ALSO BY BONNIE TSUI

*American Chinatown: A People's History
of Five Neighborhoods*

WHY WE SWIM

Why We Swim

Bonnie Tsui

ALGONQUIN BOOKS
OF CHAPEL HILL
2020

Published by
ALGONQUIN BOOKS OF CHAPEL HILL
Post Office Box 2225
Chapel Hill, North Carolina 27515-2225

a division of
WORKMAN PUBLISHING
225 Varick Street
New York, New York 10014

Excerpt from "Swimming" from *Wild Is the Wind: Poems* by Carl Phillips.
Copyright © 2018 by Carl Phillips. Reprinted by permission of
Farrar, Straus and Giroux.

"Morning Swim" copyright © 1965 by Maxine Kumin, from
Selected Poems, 1960–1990 by Maxine Kumin. Used by permission
of W. W. Norton & Company, Inc.

Excerpt from "The Swimming Song" reprinted by permission
of Loudon Wainwright III.

Library of Congress Cataloging-in-Publication Data

Names: Tsui, Bonnie, author. |
Algonquin Books of Chapel Hill (Firm)
Title: Why we swim / Bonnie Tsui.
Description: First Edition. | Chapel Hill, North Carolina :
Algonquin Books of Chapel Hill, 2020. |
Includes bibliographical references. | Summary: "Bonnie Tsui
looks at our love affair with the water, from evolution to
mythology, from survival and well-being, from community
swim clubs to competitive races, and she goes around the world to explore its
significance in many cultures"—Provided by publisher.
Identifiers: LCCN 2019042645 | ISBN 9781616207861 (Hardcover) | ISBN
9781643750514 (e-book)
Subjects: LCSH: Swimming.
Classification: LCC GV837 .T78 2020 | DDC 797.2/1—dc23
LC record available at https://lccn.loc.gov/2019042645

10 9 8 7 6 5 4 3 2

For Felix and Teddy, my water babies

CONTENTS

~

WHY WE SWIM

SURVIVAL

～

An old map from when this place was first settled shows monsters
everywhere, once the shore gives out . . .

—CARL PHILLIPS, "Swimming"

One night over dinner, my husband tells me a story he heard about a boat in the North Atlantic and a man who should have drowned. Late on the evening of March 11, 1984, a fishing trawler was working on calm seas three miles east of the island of Heimaey, part of an archipelago off the south coast of Iceland. The sky was clear, the air a wintry twenty-eight degrees Fahrenheit. There were five crew aboard the vessel. Guðlaugur Friðþórsson, the boat's mate, was just twenty-two years old; he had taken a break and was asleep below deck when he was woken up by the cook, who told him the trawling gear had snagged on the sea bottom. Soon after Friðþórsson arrived on deck, he saw that the crew were trying to winch up the gear. One of the trawl wires was taut over the side, pulling the boat over so far that the sea had begun to wash through the railings. Friðþórsson shouted a warning. The captain, Hjörtur Jónsson, gave instructions to slacken the winch, but then it jammed. A swell ran under the boat, overturning it, and the sailors found themselves pitched into the freezing sea.

Two of the men drowned almost immediately, but the remaining three, including Friðþórsson, managed to grab hold of the boat's keel. The vessel quickly began to sink, and they could not release the emergency raft. In the forty-one-degree water, they would have less than half an hour before hypothermia claimed them. The three began to swim toward the shore. Within minutes, only two remained: Jónsson and Friðþórsson.

The two men called to one other as they swam, to spur each other on. Then Jónsson stopped responding. Friðþórsson, wearing blue work pants, a red flannel shirt, and a thin sweater, kept swimming, and found himself talking to seagulls to stay awake. A boat came within three hundred and fifty feet of him and he shouted as loud as he could, but it sailed away. He swam backstroke, his eyes trained on the lighthouse at the southern end of the island. Eventually he heard the surf crashing on the coast. He prayed he would not get obliterated on the rocks. He found himself up against the base of a steep cliff, exhausted and terribly thirsty, unable to feel any of his extremities. With no way to climb up, he turned back to the sea, adjusted course, and swam farther south, where he came ashore and made his way slowly across a spiky, snow-covered lava field over a mile into town, stopping to punch through an inch-thick layer of ice on a sheep cistern to get a drink of water. When he finally arrived in town, it seemed to him a splendid dream-vision of life; he knocked on the door of the first home he saw with lights on. He was barefoot and covered in frost. Behind him was a trail of bloody footprints on the sidewalk leading up to the house.

This is a true story. In the end, Friðþórsson survived six hours in frigid seas and swam more than three and a half miles to land. When he arrived at the hospital, doctors were unable to discern his pulse. And yet he showed no signs of hypothermia, only dehydration.

Friðþórsson's body, it turns out, resembled a seal's. Researchers later determined that he was insulated by fourteen millimeters of fat—two or three times the normal human thickness, and more solid. This man was more marine mammal than terrestrial. He had a biological quirk that saved him: it kept him warm, buoyant, and able to keep swimming. Many called him a real-life selkie—that half-man, half-seal figure of Icelandic and Scottish lore. To me, he is a living reminder that we are not so far removed from the sea.

As humans, we walk the earth. We are land creatures with an aquatic past. I'm drawn to stories like Friðþórsson's because I want to know what remains of that past, today. In a way, all swimming stories—from the naiads of Greek myth to the long-distance swimmer Diana Nyad, who swam from Cuba to Florida in 2013—are attempts to reacquaint our land-adapted selves with water. We humans are not natural-born swimmers, but we have figured out ways to reclaim abilities that existed before that land-sea split in our evolution, hundreds of millions of years ago.

Why do we swim, when evolution has shaped us to excel on land by running down prey until it drops from exhaustion?

Of course it has to do with survival: Somewhere along the way, swimming helped us to get from one prehistoric lakeshore to another and escape predators of our own; to dive for that trove of bigger shellfish and get to new sources of food; to venture across oceans and settle new lands; to navigate all manner of aquatic perils and see swimming as a source of joy, pleasure, achievement. To arrive at this day, to talk about why we swim.

This book is an investigation of what seduces us to water, despite its dangers, and why we come back to it again and again. It's clear to me that once we can swim for survival, swimming can be so much more. The act of swimming can be one of healing, and health—a way to well-being. Swimming together can be a way to find community, through a team, a club, or a shared, beloved body of water. We have only to watch each other in water to know that it creates the space for play. If we get good enough at the thing, it can be an engine of competition—a way to test our mettle, in the pool or open water. Swimming is about the mind, too. To find rhythm in the water is to discover a new way of being in the world, through flow. This is about our human relationship to water and how immersion can open our imaginations.

More than 70 percent of the planet is covered by water; 40 percent of the global population lives less than sixty miles from the coast. This book is for swimmers and curious humans of every stripe and age, whether you are drawn to water for speed or distance or transcendence. This is for those who heed the siren call of the water. It's also for those of us who seek to understand ourselves, that lost, quiet state of *just being*—no technology, no beeps—dating back to our watery human origins.

We choose to put ourselves in all kinds of waters: oceans, lakes, rivers, streams, pools. We even have a romance with lifeguards, the custodians of those places. At the intersection of these things, my family story begins—and not just because my mother and father met in a swimming pool in Hong Kong.

I learned to swim when I was five years old, for the simple reason that my parents didn't want me to drown: in the bath, in the neighbor's backyard pool, at the beach. As a kid at Jones Beach, New York, I spent a lot of time in the four feet of water at the scalloped, lacy edge of the Atlantic. I can picture the scene clearly: My brother and cousins and I bob up and down in the shallows, waiting for a wave to come and lift us off our feet. We use our arms as rudders to pilot us along the face of a wave as it breaks, depositing us at the foamy intersection where water meets sand. Get up, laugh, repeat.

We are mesmerized by that heaving body of water. So is everybody else. On a hot day, and on a holiday, a hundred thousand other people might be there at Jones Beach. Lifeguards sit sentinel at their elevated stations, policing the crowds from behind mirrored sunglasses.

There's something primal about a day like that at the beach—it's all the animals heading to the watering hole. Water is a magnet for our teeming throng of humanity. I watch the ways people dip in and out. Some are just there to cool off: electrifying entry, quick exit. Some stay awhile, floating and splashing and swimming. Always there are people who keep their distance and don't go in at all. But still they come, hypnotized by the pulse of the ocean, alive to the sound of the surf and the smell of the briny air.

I felt the draw of liquid early on: that slide into lovely immersion, that spiraling weightlessness, that privileged access to a muted underworld. Entry was granted to me there at Jones Beach, where we passed the hours within shouting distance of our moms' blue-flowered beach towels. In between swims, we gave each other wedgies and buried ourselves in the sand. I liked how the ocean seemed to draw breath, lying placid one moment and rearing up the next, moving us in one rippling mass to and from the horizon. Once, a big wave came and smacked me from behind. Surprise overturning, ass over teakettle. Then, a liquid, green room, clouded by sand. Me, swimming and swimming toward nothing. *Which way is up?* Four feet isn't very much water, but it's deep enough to drown in.

Time stretched. I wondered about the press of my burning lungs, wishing for air.

Time restarted with an accidental kick to the head, from my cousin swimming not two feet away. Gifted this reference point, I scrambled to the surface, my hair wrapped around my face like kelp. Embarrassed and gasping, I looked around. When I realized that no one had noticed I was in trouble, I pretended that I never was. And I turned right back into the sea.

What could bring on this voluntary amnesia? What did I find so alluring about the water that I could forgive a murder attempt by the sea, and so quickly at that? Most every year, a handful of people drown at the beaches of Long Island. At the time, I was just a young swimmer, going back for more of the magic: the illusion of being native to an element that is not home to humans like me.

What I experienced that day stayed with me—three decades later I'm an adult who swims for pleasure and exercise nearly every day, and yet I wonder about the deeper, more primitive instincts that drive us. We are pulled to the paradox of water as a source of life and death, and we have figured out myriad ways to conduct ourselves in it. Not everybody is a swimmer, but everyone has a swimming story to tell. In the examination of this universal experience—and it is universal, whether you are fearful of the water or not; whether you love it or leave it, you will encounter it at some point in your life—we find ourselves flexing our survival muscles, achieving something quietly triumphant with our persistence in the medium. Together we are pool-hopping, chasing oases, immersing ourselves, in search of the bait that pulls us into the depths. This is an exploration of a world. Let's go for a swim.

We begin with a shellfish.

1

Stone Age Swimming

The abalone does not want to come off the rock. Fifteen feet underwater, I jab the metal abalone iron underneath the shell, between the mollusk's muscular foot and the boulder it's fastened to, hoping for the pop I've been promised. Nothing.

I try again, my breath beginning to bubble out of my nose with the effort of swimming in place, fighting the currents that are pulling me to and fro. Still nothing. This abalone, evidently sensing my presence, has locked down tight. Once that happens, I am finding, it is nearly impossible to remove.

Diving for abalone is an attractive but dangerous sport. In pursuit of the elusive mollusk, I've submerged myself in the waters of Salt Point State Park, along the solitary, switchbacked Sonoma Coast two and a half hours north of San Francisco. The hazards are many: cold water, rip currents, rocks, kelp tangles, heavy surf, sharks. Still, most every season, April through November, thousands of hopeful swimmers make their way to the Northern California coast to try their hand at abalone hunting. The wild red abalone is the biggest in the world and is found only on the west coast of North America. It's where I can play the role of prehistoric hunter, swimming down for my dinner, with zero experience.

I hold a scuba certification, but over the years all that gear has come to feel claustrophobic and encumbering when I'm in the water. Here on this part of the coast, scuba tanks are illegal, so abalone divers are armed with few tools beyond their breath-holding and swimming skills. The reality of this back-to-basics, man-versus-nature pursuit is that every cove along this part of the coast, rangers say, is a gravesite: in 2015, four people died while abalone diving during the first three weeks of the season alone. It turns out that even experienced divers can't hold their breath for long; people who are used to wearing full tanks of air start to panic when confronted with this fact. In the murky water, it's tough to stay oriented. The swell will toss you against the rocks and then suck you out to sea.

But still, I want to try. I learn to spot the abalone's rippling lip of black tissue, or mantle, against the side of a big, craggy escarpment. I struggle to dislodge one, then another. An ancient, pea-size part of my brain lights up with satisfaction when I jackknife down to the seafloor, eyes on the prize, and finally hoist a six-pound abalone out of the water. I need both hands to haul it up and both legs to propel me; I can feel the grin forming on my lips before my head even breaks the surface.

I've never felt the urge to shoot a bird for breakfast or run down a deer for dinner. But the direct appeal of swimming for my lunch is clear from the moment I spy the shellfish. There is something I need to understand about the act of swimming for something more essential than exercise. In my backyard later that day, I clean, trim, and pound the meat tender—yep, with a rock—cook it up over a flame, and feed my family of four a meal I've prepared entirely with my own hands and breath and body. We are divorced from our food sources; it is a recognized symptom of modern life. Swimming for resources allows me, for a moment, to resolve the disconnect. That evening, when I rinse my hands in the sink and watch the water drain away, I remember the rhythmic sluicing of seawater through the rocks along the shoreline and what it felt like to watch it all flow back toward the horizon.

THE FIRST KNOWN record of swimming lies in the middle of a desert. Somewhere in Egypt, near the Libyan border, in the Sahara's remote and mountainous Gilf Kebir plateau, there are swimmers breaststroking up the walls of a cave.

The Cave of Swimmers, discovered by the Hungarian explorer László Almásy in 1933, contains a trove of Neolithic paintings that depict people in a range of underwater poses. Archaeologists have dated the creation of the artwork as far back as ten thousand years ago. At the time of Almásy's discovery, the notion that the Sahara had not always been a desert was a radical idea. Theories of a climate change that could account for the shift from temperate environs to barren, hyper-arid desert were so new that the editor of Almásy's 1934 book, *The Unknown Sahara*, reportedly felt compelled to insert footnotes stating disagreement. But the paintings convinced Almásy himself that water might have been a natural feature in the immediate vicinity of the cave, that the swimmers themselves were the painters, that a lake lapped their very toes as they worked. Where there is now a sea of sand, there was water flowing. Where one medium is liquid life, the other may seem to be its parched, granular antithesis, he thought, but the two were indeed connected.

It turns out, of course, that Almásy was right. Decades later, archaeologists would find dried lake beds not far from the cave, from a time when the Sahara was green. His answer to the riddle of swimmers in the desert would eventually be confirmed with a remarkable abundance of geological evidence showing a landscape once dotted with ancient lakes, as well as the startling discovery of hippo bones and the remains of many other water-dwelling animals, including giant tortoises, fish, and clams. This wet period became known as the Green Sahara.

Not long ago, in an old issue of *National Geographic*, I read about a paleontologist named Paul Sereno who further confirmed Almásy's hunch. In the fall of 2000, Sereno was hunting for dinosaur bones in a different part of the Sahara, the southern edge, in conflict-prone, little-explored Niger. In the open desert, some 125 miles from the country's largest city,

Agadez, one of his expedition photographers scrambled up a remote group of dunes—and stumbled across a massive trove of skeletons. This time, the bones weren't from dinosaurs or hippos.

These eroding, windswept sand dunes revealed what turned out to be hundreds of human remains, interspersed with prehistoric fragments of pottery that were up to ten thousand years old. Some of the pottery pieces were carved with wavy lines; others were stippled with dots. The burial place, which the scientists called Gobero, the Tuareg tribal name for the area, was the largest and earliest Stone Age cemetery found to date. It turns out that the Green Sahara was exactly the sort of place where prehistoric human swimmers might exist.

ON A BITINGLY cold January afternoon, I meet Paul Sereno at his fossil lab at the University of Chicago, where he has been a professor for more than thirty years. There isn't much scholarship specific to Stone Age swimming, so I want him to help me conjure up a picture of this prehistoric world. Sereno doesn't swim much himself, but he has spent a lot of time thinking about the swimming abilities of both dinosaurs and people (he's one of the scientists whose research established *Spinosaurus aegyptiacus* as the first known swimming dinosaur). There's a dash of Indiana Jones to him—he has the leather jacket and the restless enthusiasm, and he was once voted one of *People* magazine's "50 Most Beautiful People."

I ask Sereno to reconstruct for me an ancient environment that was suitable for swimming. In the Green Sahara of ten thousand years ago, he says, Gobero resembled "a Daytona Beach in the desert"—a vast interlinked system of shallow lakes, many of them about ten feet deep, with sand spits that allowed humans to walk out to the water.

Scientists have named the aquatic system Paleolake Gobero. One of its most critical geographic features was a fault on one side, which did two things. One, it dammed up deep ground-water, so there was always water there even if it didn't rain for a long while. Two, when it did rain, or when the ground-water welled up, the fault cliff acted as a natural dam flanking the site, with periodic spills to regulate levels in the basin. The shallow aquatic system came and went, but it was stable enough that people lived along its shores for many thousands of years. The pristine burial site contained the remains of two distinct populations of humans, their occupations separated by a period of a thousand years, during which the lake disappeared and the site was abandoned. This greening and drying of the Sahara, Sereno says, was the largest climate change since the last ice age, about twelve thousand years ago.

There were immense middens of shucked clamshells—so many shells that Sereno thinks the people of Gobero must have dived for clams as well as collected them from shore. And the evidence there suggests that this was not the only means of catching dinner. There were carved fishhooks and finely honed barbed harpoon tips made from the jawbones of crocodiles. Sereno and his team even found four harpoons embedded in the lake bed itself. "They likely had boats," Sereno says. "But we have no idea what the boats looked like, or what they were made of. And with the harpoons way out in the middle of the lake bed, I'd guess that they probably swam with their boats, too."

Sereno's team also discovered heavy, flat-bottomed stones—what they suspect to be weights for netting fish like tilapia and catfish. In a lab workroom where researchers clean and prepare materials for display, he hands me one of these, a smooth, brown-speckled oval that has a pleasing heft. In that lake, the ancient fishermen speared and landed impressive catches of Nile perch, a freshwater monstrosity that can grow to six feet long and weigh more than four hundred pounds. The species, though in decline today, is still an important food source in many parts of Africa.

A lot of things surprise me as I poke about the lab of this famous paleontologist. Sereno is pretty blithe about the test tubes of invaluable early human DNA bagged up and sitting on his desk (still waiting to be sent out for analysis) and about the half-prepped new dinosaur species in his cabinet (still waiting to be named). If you have a roaming curiosity that refuses to settle long enough to get hung up on paperwork, I suppose you'd leave those things lying around, too.

"Have you ever seen a dinosaur mummy? I love mummies!" he exclaims as he invites me to examine a rare dinosaur fossil that reveals the specimen's textured hide. I run my fingers lightly over the imprint's bumps and ridges. The first thing that comes to my mind is *dinosaur leather*, and I can't stop myself from blurting it out loud. Sereno allows me to handle everything in the lab—from sharp arrowheads and fragile pottery to a plate from a stegosaurus and *even the remnants of a T. rex*. This physical proximity to the past, paired with Sereno's enthusiastic, mile-a-minute commentary, is nothing short of spellbinding. A little side trip to Prehistoric Times.

But, with all the evidence, we still can't tell how well the people of Paleolake Gobero swam—the frustrating thing about investigating the trail of humans' aquatic past is that a wake doesn't stick around. What Sereno and his researchers can show is that these inhabitants of the Green Sahara led a hunter-gatherer existence, pool-hopping as needed but mostly staying put by the water.

I like to imagine that these early humans dove for their towers of clams the way I dove for abalone—with some kicking and bobbing and gasping, yes, but also with a measure of wonder and joy. It's not so hard to picture how that might have happened. I think about my own sons, who are no happier than when it's low tide in Bolinas, a little coastal hamlet an hour north of where we live in Berkeley, California. In the mornings, there's often a low fog hanging over the silvery lagoon. The boys race around on the muddy flats revealed by the receding tide, leaping over darkly sandy rivulets. They dart to and from the edge of a restless ocean. They throw seaweed at each other. They build pyramids of sand, jabbering a detailed backstory to go with the miniature complex they have constructed, before they inundate the whole thing with a mass flood. I watch as they dance in and out of the water, continually testing their comfort with the depths. They both love the sea. Felix, the older, has known how to swim for some time, but Teddy, the younger, is still shy around water that moves of its own accord.

Perhaps it happened this same way, so many thousands of years ago. A girl gathers clams at the edge of a paleolake. It's been her job as long as she can remember. She can see the clams just beyond the drop-off to deeper waters. Maybe those clams are bigger than the ones she can reach just by wading. One day, she wonders if she could hold her breath to get to them. Little by little, she ventures out and back, out and back, pushing off the sandy bottom with her toes, bobbing at the surface, frog kicking her legs to free her face from the water. Weeks go by, maybe months. The bobbing and gasping eventually give way to something she can sustain. She knows what it is to float untroubled, conserving energy, and what it is to scissor her body and swoop down when she spies a promising mollusk. She finds success in unearthing a new cache of food. Others start to imitate her up-down, up-down method.

There's a magic to being able to look at tangible objects from a bygone era—to say, *See here. They were here, where we stand, right now.* To point at a curved arm bracelet made of hippo ivory and say, *She wore this.* To pick up the jagged tip of a spear and picture those water hunters diving and digging and swimming. *Paleo man! Just like us!*

These early humans were agile enough to avoid hippos and crocodiles that shared the water with them, and they would have had time enough to master swimming, because they weren't scouring the landscape in search of water or food. The lake, and the animal riches contained therein, made it possible for these societies to thrive for millennia right on its shores. Elsewhere in the Green Sahara, during this same wet period, perhaps those cave painters were swimming, too.

Though the earliest evidence of human swimming dates back just ten thousand years, we most likely knew how to swim much earlier than that. Our modern human species, *Homo sapiens*, began to evolve nearly two hundred thousand years ago from other species of now-extinct ancestral humans. There is evidence of those ancestral humans going to sea, too. In 2008, on the Greek island of Crete, a team of researchers found quartz stone hand axes that were hundreds of thousands of years old, embedded in rock terraces near cave shelters on the southern coast. The rough tools were unlike any others previously found there and resembled those used by *Homo erectus*, a species of ancestral human found in Africa and mainland Europe. Because Crete has been separated from the mainland for five million years, those ancestral humans would have had to travel to the island by open water. It was proof of Mediterranean seafaring peoples tens of thousands of years earlier than scientists had previously thought. Open-ocean voyages are pretty hard to pull off if you don't know how to swim, or if you don't have comfort and familiarity with the water.

Even Neanderthals, extinct close relatives of humans, may have swum for their food. I consult the British anthropologist Chris Stringer, who studies Neanderthals and is an expert on human origins at London's Natural History Museum; his team's findings from caves in Gibraltar showed that late-surviving Neanderthals, who overlapped with modern humans, lived off the sea about twenty-eight thousand years ago, before they died out. The Neanderthals collected mussels from a river estuary and butchered seals and dolphins, dragging them into caves for food prep by the fire. How did Neanderthals catch those fish and dolphins and seals? We can't tell if or how they swam, but the distribution of the marine animal remains in the caves' strata shows that Neanderthals had longtime knowledge and familiarity with coastal resources, a behavior that has rarely been found before modern humans came along.

But if diving for abalone taught me anything, it is how easy the act of swimming can seem—and how imperceptible the dangers can be. Sereno tells me that the most striking discovery at Gobero actually has to do with swimming, and drowning: a moving triple burial at the edge of the paleolake that his team dubbed the "Stone Age Embrace."

He describes what it was like to uncover the three bodies: a thirty-year-old woman and two small children, aged five and eight, lying intimately together with hands intertwined.

"It was a spectacular burial, three crania coming to the surface," he says, recalling the delicate unearthing of the skulls. The team moved carefully during the excavation, which was difficult to perform. Loose sand moves like water; every time you brush it away, it trickles back.

The poignancy of the pose—arms stretched to the other, holding hands—affected everyone on the expedition. The arrangement seemed clearly ceremonial, Sereno says. A sample of sand taken at the scene later showed that flowers—a species in a genus called *Celosia*, part of the amaranth family, that can come in many colors—had been laid down. Arrowheads carved from petrified wood were found underneath the bodies. They were X-rayed and scanned with an electron microscope: the analysis showed that they were never fired, and were probably deliberately placed there for symbolic purposes. When examined, the skeletons and teeth revealed no stress patterns of injury or disease.

Sereno asks me if I'd like to meet the people of Gobero. Right now. He leads me to the excavated display of the triple burial, pointing out the arrowheads, the healthy teeth, the deliberate placement of the bodies. Though being in the presence of so many tangible paleontological finds—the dinosaurs, the other ancient aquatic animals—was profound, I found the encounter with the human remains to be even more so. I realized that it's the story embedded in the earth with them that captivates me most. The Stone Age embrace is at heart a story familiar to you and me: the three (a mother and her children?) died together, suddenly (drowning?), and someone (a loving husband and father?) had time to perform an elaborate burial ritual.

Sereno confirms at least some of my imaginings. "When can you pose a body? You have to contend with rigor mortis and rotting in the sun," he explains. "So it was a sudden death somehow. On water's edge. I think it was the result of drowning in Paleolake Gobero."

It is a timeless tale of a parent's worst nightmare. I know what it is to be that child on the beach, playing and exploring. And I know now what it is like to be a parent, watching my two young sons learn to swim and experiment by the water. Then as now, the states of swimming and drowning are terrifyingly, thrillingly porous. It remains that way no matter how well we have mastered the skill.

Wet periods punctuated by long dry ones also allowed pieces of that past to persist to this day, for us to find. Collapsed into the tragedy of the triple burial is the beginning of everything; another timeless tale, of course, is that of a drowned world. A cyclical variation in Earth's orbit brought Africa's seasonal monsoons north and made the Green Sahara possible; Gobero is an unparalleled record of the humans who lived there. The remnants of these lives have special resonance for us today, when waters are rising higher and temperatures are fluctuating above and beyond what we have ever recorded.

We ourselves may soon be devastated by water, and this time our own activities are the cause of dramatic changes to the surface of the planet. By 2030, the number of people affected by floods is expected to triple. In California, where I live, sea level rise could exceed nine feet by the turn of the next century, washing away more than 50 percent of the beaches of the Golden State. Worldwide, sea level rise has the potential to turn hundreds of millions of people into refugees.

2

You're a Land Animal

Most land mammals possess instinctive swimming ability from birth, but humans do not. Elephants, dogs, cats (albeit reluctantly), and even bats can swim (and pretty well, too). Humans and other large primates, like chimpanzees, have to be taught. Some scientists speculate that this has to do with the way the anatomy of the great apes evolved to be better suited to swinging through trees. In the rare experimental cases in which apes were taught to swim by researchers, they exhibited a froglike kick, instead of the doggy paddle so common in other mammals.

You evolved from fish, Paul Sereno tells me, but now "you're a land animal trying to swim. You're what we call a secondary swimmer."

Don't be too disappointed just yet. The paleobiologist Neil Shubin explains that the structure of the human body is the legacy of ancient fish, reptiles, and other primates. In a 2014 documentary based on his book *Your Inner Fish*, Shubin says that "being a fish paleontologist is a very powerful way to teach human anatomy, because often some of the best road maps to our own bodies are seen in other creatures." The fish's legacy: their fins, our limbs, all start from the same group of cells.

Within us there are intriguing traces of a swimming past. And if we hold in our bodies the ghosts of other animals, it follows that hints of certain functions remain and reawaken with submersion. If you put a two-month-old facedown in water, the baby will hold her breath for several seconds and her heart rate will slow, conserving oxygen. But that doesn't mean she'll swim to safety if you throw her in a pool. As babies get older and their neurological systems develop, that bradycardic reflex—part of a whole suite of primitive or residual reflexes that include sucking and grasping—starts to weaken.

Humans, though, are imitation machines. We learn through observation: everything from movement patterns to reading the emotions of people we encounter, in domains ranging from tool-making and food preferences to ideas about fairness, mating, and language. "The key to understanding how humans evolved and why we are so different from other animals is to recognize that we are a cultural species," writes the evolutionary biologist Joseph Henrich, whose influential work centers on how cultural and genetic evolution interact. Cumulative social learning—our ability to form large-scale "collective brains," as Henrich calls it—is particular to us. Other animals exhibit social learning, but humans are singular in doing it on a cumulative cultural level that actually influences genetic evolution.

Henrich illustrates his theory with case studies from his cheekily named "Lost European Explorer Files": When European explorers got marooned in some new, seemingly inhospitable environment—the Arctic, say, or Australia— they invariably died of starvation, sickness, or exposure, except in the cases when they fell in with local indigenous peoples. Those locals were robust and healthy; they knew how to thrive in the so-called harsh environment and had for millennia. Human groups connect and build bodies of knowledge that no single individual is smart enough to figure out in one lifetime: how to make a triple-barbed fishing spear, what to burn for fire in the absence of wood, how to leach poisons out of a toxic plant to make it edible. Paleoarchaeological records indicate that this kind of cultural evolution has been happening for at least the last two hundred and eighty thousand years—and that it rapidly accelerated over the last ten thousand of those.

This culture-gene coevolution helps explain the outstanding evolutionary success our species has had on our planet. Individually, we aren't all that special or smart. But our ability to acquire, store, organize, and pass on an ever-growing body of information over generations makes us smarter than any one person or group. The practice of swimming, and the different ways in which we teach ourselves to swim, is part of that collective cultural knowledge. When it comes to swimming, it is not just the how-to—the formal instruction—that is critical but also the ways we communicate the importance of that knowledge, through the stories we tell.

A brief history of what we have come up with to aid us in swimming over the last two millennia or so:

~400 BC, Rome: a cork life jacket, described by Plutarch and worn by a messenger sent by the Roman general Camillus to swim the Tiber because the bridge was in the possession of the Gauls.

Fourteenth-century Persia: the translucent outer layer of a tortoise shell, to protect the eyes while diving for pearls.

Fifteenth-century Italy: a bladder constructed of animal skin and blown full of air, for breathing underwater, designed by Leonardo da Vinci, who also made sketches for swim fins, a snorkel, and other buoyancy devices.

Date unknown, Japan: a rope line attached to a pulley, used by the *ama*—Japanese free-diving fisherwomen—to reel themselves up from the depths in case of swimming or breathing troubles.

1702, Boston: swim paddles in the shape of oval painters' palettes to wear on the hands, from inventor and expert waterman Benjamin Franklin, to go faster.

1896, elsewhere in Massachusetts: a metal-framed "swimming machine" to hold a student safely in the water, with mechanical arm and leg supports that moved the body in the appropriate stroke and kick motion, patented by James Emerson.

1908, London: a set of water-wings sewn from fine cotton material, with valves for inflation—tens of thousands were sold to the public under the brand Swimeesy Buoy.

1930, Miami: a wooden swimming costume fashioned from thin strips of spruce, a novelty to encourage and keep timid female swimmers afloat.

2017, China: a tiny handheld device with double propellers, the WhiteShark Mix, promises to help any beginner "swim like a champion and become an uncontested star in the water."

Sometimes we need a little help. If the complement to human biology is culture, then our strength is our ability to identify a problem and invent the solution. The names of these inventions and their descriptions are for me a kind of aquatic poetry. It is the sound of our imaginations dancing with our biology to make the impossible possible.

3

Lessons from a Sea Nomad

I n the coastal regions of Southeast Asia's Coral Triangle, we get a glimpse of swimming lessons in a vanishing aquatic society. The best free-diving fishermen can swim down to two hundred feet and stay there, alternately swimming and walking along the ocean floor—humans are negatively buoyant at that depth—spear guns in hand, for ten minutes at a time, until they find their prey. They can spend five hours a day submerged underwater.

For thousands of years, in what is today Malaysia, Indonesia, and the Philippines, the youngest Bajau sea nomads have been initiated into a life of the sea before they even learn to walk. Parents pray that babies will be blessed with the aquatic abilities they need for a life joined with the reef. Even two- and three-year-olds can dive with ease, their legs flicking powerfully to propel them to collect small clams. From their families' houseboats, older children teach their younger siblings how to float and kick and look for fish.

The Bajau have recently been shown to have spleens that are 50 percent larger than those of a related group of villagers on the Indonesian mainland. When we dive underwater, the spleen contracts as part of the mammalian diving reflex, shooting its supply of oxygenated red blood cells into circulation around the body. The heart rate slows, and blood vessels constrict, directing blood flow away from the extremities and toward major organs. These energy conservation measures kick in so we can use available oxygen more efficiently.

Marine mammals such as seals, who spend much of their lives underwater, have disproportionately large spleens compared with land-based mammals. Seals with the largest spleens can dive deepest—think of it as having an extra tank of air. Research shows that the Bajau's oversize spleens are due to natural selection, not to diving itself: Bajau people with genes that produce larger spleens tend to survive and have more offspring. Even Bajau who have never been divers have the same trait. Their bodies have evolved to be better at free diving.

Though this particular trait of the Bajau is inherited, other aquatic characteristics are acquired. Similar free-diving sea nomads, like the water-dwelling Moken—who also live on houseboats and coastal homes on stilts, in communities throughout what is today Thailand and Myanmar—have a special ability to focus their eyes underwater. The Moken kids who grow up diving have been shown to have underwater vision that is twice as sharp as that of us landlubbers. Where the rest of us see a blur, these mer-people can easily gather clams and sea cucumbers from the ocean floor without the aid of goggles or masks.

Most of us see terribly underwater because the refractive power of the curved cornea, which works so well on land, is offset by immersion in water. Sea nomad kids are able to accommodate for that when they are underwater by constricting their pupils, which increases the fine detail of what they can see. At first, it wasn't clear whether this ability was inherited or learned. But researchers figured out that early immersion training can change all of us. In fewer than a dozen visual practice sessions aimed at distinguishing specific kinds of contrasting patterns underwater, non-sea-nomad kids were able to achieve a lasting heightened ability to focus underwater.

The water has shaped these peoples in other ways, too. Survival in these places requires not just swimming skills but also an understanding of how the aquatic environment works. These cultures take steps to prepare themselves. On December 26, 2004, when a massive tsunami in the Indian Ocean killed some two hundred and thirty thousand people along the coastlines of South and Southeast Asia, the Moken survived by reading signs in the water.

On the remote Surin Islands off the coast of Thailand, Moken villagers fled toward higher ground after someone noticed the sea receding and the shore going dry. They warned everyone they saw and were gone long before the first wave hit. The village was decimated, but all of its residents were saved. In Mu Ko Surin National Park, some two dozen Moken were out guiding tourists on snorkeling excursions when they recognized that the currents were moving strangely; they steered their boats away from the coast into deeper water and survived. A similar thing happened to a group of Moken fishermen out in Myanmar-governed waters; after observing fiercely swirling water around their vessels, they immediately headed further out to sea. Other fishermen in the vicinity were busy with the squid harvest; when the seas rose up with a terrific violence, they were tossed to their deaths.

Elsewhere in the region, elephants stampeded for higher ground. Cicadas went silent. Dolphins swam toward the depths. None of these Moken had ever seen a tsunami them-selves, but Moken elders spoke of the legend of the "seven roller waves," which come once every two generations. *Laboon* was the name they had for the biggest of the waves—it was a "cleansing wave," one that arrived with a fury to consume and destroy.

Similar stories of sudden saltwater floods and mass drownings exist in the oral tradition of First Nations and Native American tribes in the Pacific Northwest and are con-firmed by Japanese tsunami records dating back one and a half millennia. Knowledge is encoded in these stories. Bajau legends about half-fish people and Moken stories about the seven big waves are really stories about how to live a life at sea. Over thousands of years, without a written language, storytelling is how these peoples have successfully passed along the aquatic skills so key to their longevity and survival: swimming, diving, fishing, boating, all of it made possible by keen observation and intimate knowledge of the marine environment.

The stories teach reverence. Before diving, the Bajau make an offering to the ocean spirits—a bit of food floated in a coconut-husk boat, a cigarette in a leaf, a stick of incense—because the ocean spirits can be kind or cruel. They are mercurial, and with their mood goes the mood of the frothing seas. If you are humble before them—if you are gentle with the coral, if you are respectful of the fish and don't take more than you need—the ocean will take care of you.

The last of these historically nomadic fishermen struggle today to adapt to a changing world, where, as stateless people with no citizenship, no documents, and few options for work, they are perceived by many governments as adrift in the worst sense. And yet, even as the Bajau and Moken ways of life are eroding around them—fewer and fewer are able to continue a life of subsistence fishing—the last vestiges of their culture still tell them how to swim to survive.

WE ARE NOT amphibious, but I like the idea of amphibiousness. The naturalist Loren Eiseley wrote that the great accomplishment of modern science was the ability to time travel—not just through the concrete observations of the world around us (reading "seams of exposed strata") but also through our own imaginings ("I saw the drifting cells of the early seas"). "The salt of those ancient seas is in our blood, its lime is in our bones," he wrote. "Every time we walk along

a beach some ancient urge disturbs us so that we find ourselves shedding shoes and garments, or scavenging among
seaweed and whitened timbers like the homesick refugees of
a long war." We are products of physical evolution, but we
are driven by our interpretation of that evolutionary history.

The awareness of rising seas is being built into many
modern-day societies living waterside, like the Dutch. The
swimming lessons we can take from them involve actual
swimming lessons: to earn the right to use public pools freely,
all Dutch children take classes to get a diploma that certifies
their ability to swim in their clothes and shoes.

I am riveted by a striking underwater photo of fully
clothed Dutch fifth graders in one of these swimming classes.
It makes sense—they wear garments every day, don't they?
And so if the water comes, they will be ready. It hits me that
this kind of thinking is in alignment with the traditional
adaptiveness of the sea nomads: that we should teach ourselves how to live *with* water, not how to keep it at bay.

"It's a basic part of our culture, like riding a bike," the
Dutch architect Rem Koolhaas once told the *New York
Times*. Everything is constructed and conducted with an
awareness of the possibility of flood; a national water man-
agement center controls the day-to-day flow of water in and
out of the Netherlands. The mayor of Rotterdam, Ahmed
Aboutaleb, explained that his city lies in the most vulnerable part of the country. In the case of a flood coming in and
overpowering the system they have created, "from the rivers

or the sea, we can evacuate maybe fifteen out of a hundred people," he said. "We have no choice. We must learn to live with water."

We must learn to live with water, and then it opens us up to possibility. We first swim to survive the water—we can't view swimming as anything else until that happens. But once we can survive it, the water can be something more for us. We can live with it, thrive with it. I think of Charles Tomlinson's poem "Swimming Chenango Lake," which captures this state of being. He describes swimming as the act of moving in the embrace of water, but mindfully. To do so is to realize what it means to be, as Tomlinson writes, "between grasp and grasping, free."

4

~

The Human Seal

G uðlaugur Friðþórsson learned to swim as a boy in a
public swimming pool in 1960s Iceland. His island,
Heimaey—it means "home island"—is the largest of
the Vestmannaeyjar, or Westman Islands, and its only inhabited place.

In the first of three photos he shows me from that time,
kids frolic with white foam kickboards, yet another inge-
nious swimming invention, under the watchful supervision
of an instructor stationed at the edge of the pool. In the background, behind the pool's high-walled perimeter, you can see
the craggy volcanic island topography in which the town,
also called Vestmannaeyjar, sits.

In the second photo, puffs of ominous black smoke hover
above the cool blue rectangle of the pool and its neighboring
red-roofed, white buildings. In the final photo, taken during
the volcanic eruption of 1973, there is an incandescent river
of lava flowing through town. In the end, the community
of five thousand people was evacuated by the island's fishing fleet, and this part of Guðlaugur's hometown—including

his old pool—fell victim to the lava. (In Iceland, people are known and addressed by their first names, the surname being simply whose son or daughter you are, a convention I will apply throughout this chapter.) A new swimming hall, built with donations after the eruption, would feature a series of pools heated with the resulting geothermal energy.

The 1973 eruption is notable because Iceland decided to fight the lava—to halt the fiery flow with massive hoses pumping cold seawater—to save the harbor. Heimaey is one of the most important fishing centers in Iceland, with a critical harbor situated along the south coast. Today, its fishing boats still account for about 15 percent of the country's fish catch by volume. Though lava engulfed much of the town, it actually improved the harbor upon which the island, and Iceland itself, depends, narrowing its mouth and making it more protected from rough weather. It gave Heimaey millions of tons of ash for paving the streets, geothermal heat that warmed the town's buildings for a decade, and a new conical volcano to go with the one the island already had. It also increased the size of the island by 20 percent, creating steep new cliffs over a hundred feet high. Near the base of these inhospitable, wave-battered cliffs, on the east side of the island, is the place where Guðlaugur came ashore in the wee hours of March 12, 1984.

Guðlaugur himself is viewed as emblematic of the national character of Iceland. The writer John McPhee immortalized the people of Iceland in the *New Yorker* thusly: "No matter how overwhelming a situation might seem to be, if there was any possibility of fighting back they had done so, and this seemed to have produced evolutionary effects, expressed in the battle against the lava, and much confirmed in the following story." The story that McPhee went on to tell, as you might guess, is Guðlaugur's. Note the language: *evolutionary effects.* It's a way to say that Icelanders are a people apart, that they are extraordinary in their hardiness, that they claim Guðlaugur as exemplary of what they hold dear.

It's a heavy load, being Iceland's epic symbol of survival and resilience. A friend who works in the fishing industry tells me that his Icelandic colleagues vividly remember the day in 1984 when Guðlaugur's fishing vessel went down. People make pilgrimages to see where Guðlaugur hit land, where he had to turn back into the water to swim to the place where he could climb across the razor-sharp lava fields into town. At times, he had to crawl on all fours. The basin he drank from so desperately is still there, marked in multiple languages. How much of his story is still remembered by Icelanders? "All of it," they say.

For a people living on a speck of land in the sea, Guðlaugur is heroic because, well, he reminds them of heroic tales: In an Icelandic saga dating back to the year 1300, there is the outlaw Grettir the Strong, who swam seven kilometers from the island of Drangey to the mainland. When he arrived, he warmed himself in a hot pool that is still there. Icelandic history is a ledger of lives lost at sea, sometimes just a few yards offshore. Heimaey's longtime importance as a fishing port means that its tiny population has disproportionately weathered the blow. An entire wall of Vestmannaeyjar's history museum is given over to records, dating back to the year 1251, of drowning incidents off the island's coast. As a result, the island has been a pioneer in swimming education and in the development of boat safety equipment: rubber life rafts, safety belts, rescue suits. Swimming lessons became routine in Vestmannaeyjar's harbor in 1891 and were held there until the town's first pool was built, in 1934. In 1943, swimming instruction was made mandatory in all of Iceland's schools. For Vestmannaeyjar, the year 2003 was distinctive because no one drowned.

Guðlaugur survived his ordeal for two critical reasons—because he occupies the body that he does, *and* because he is a good swimmer. One or the other alone would not have sufficed. In the annals of extraordinary real-life swims, Guðlaugur's is special. To me, his story is a unique intertwining of human biology and culture.

The scientific experimentation Guðlaugur later underwent with a team of Icelandic and British scientists—who determined his unusual ability to retain a nearly normal core body temperature in extreme cold water, contributing to our medical understanding of hypothermia—made him famous the world over. Even my mother-in-law, who at the time was an operating-room nurse in Massachusetts, read about his case in a medical journal. Reporters called Guðlaugur "the human seal." A few months after the accident, the international media had tracked him down while he was visiting with friends in the United States, and *The Tonight Show with*

Johnny Carson called. He turned to his friends and told them it was time for him to go back to Iceland.

For someone who is so mythic in Iceland—in this country of three hundred and thirty thousand people, there was a time when he was as famous as Björk—Guðlaugur is resolutely off the radar. Now in his mid-fifties and married, he still lives on Heimaey. He has two daughters and five grandchildren. For a time he returned to sea as a fisherman, but for many years now he has worked as an engineer at a large fish processing plant on the island. As a general rule, he no longer talks to journalists, deeply uncomfortable with the attention that the press has brought him over the past three decades.

Our correspondence begins when I decide to write him a letter anyway. I send it via registered mail; over three weeks, I track its progress across the Atlantic. *A wing and a prayer*, I think. One afternoon, I get the alert that the letter has arrived at its destination in Vestmannaeyjar. The next morning, in my inbox, I receive an e-mail from Guðlaugur.

In 2012, the Icelandic director Baltasur Kormákur, who is best known internationally for big-budget action films starring the likes of Mark Wahlberg and Denzel Washington, made a movie about Guðlaugur. Baltasur himself was a teenager when Guðlaugur's fishing vessel capsized, but as it has for his fellow Icelanders, the memory looms large. "Like everyone else in our small country, I felt for all the people of the Westman Islands who again had lost men at sea, but I was also fascinated by the news on the sole survivor," Baltasur told a British newspaper. "Who was this man? What was he made of?"

Guðlaugur was unhappy with the renewed scrutiny that the film brought. He had finally begun to settle into a life out of the spotlight, but the movie yanked him back in. "Make the movie when I'm dead," he'd told the filmmakers when they approached him. I appreciate his reticence and his resistance to fame. I also understand the global fascination. We are captivated by survival stories because we hope they will reveal something about human nature in extremis. Remember *Robinson Crusoe*, one of the most well-known of all survival tales; the author, Daniel Defoe, wrote of his interest in what emerges of one's character under duress: "I am most entertained with those Actions which give me a Light into the Nature of Man."

Guðlaugur is a man of few words, something that I gather from our e-mail correspondence. But there are glimmers of insight in his letters that intrigue me in the manner that Defoe describes. Swimming saves lives, Guðlaugur tells me; there is freedom in that. And so I get on a flight to Iceland to meet him in person.

ON A COLD, diamond-bright afternoon in March, I arrive in Heimaey on a tiny red-and-white propeller plane. On our approach, we fly through a low-lying sea mist; I peer out the window to watch the island's twin volcanic cones emerge, the dramatic, undulating landscape suddenly real and three-dimensional. From town, I can see the series of turquoise-blue buildings down in the harbor where Guðlaugur works. The mythic swimmer with whom I have been corresponding for a year, and whom I have been thinking about for much longer, is here, and he's a real guy who uses Facebook. *(Mythic swimmers: just like us.)* We make a date to meet the next evening after work.

I've planned my visit for March so I can attend what's called Guðlaugssund, or "Guðlaugur's swim." In a tradition begun by the local navigation college, there is a 6-kilometer (3.7-mile) swimming event held in Guðlaugur's honor and for those lost at sea. Year in and year out, ever since the first anniversary of the accident, the citizens of Vestmannaeyjar have faithfully carried out Guðlaugssund. In the first two decades of the swim, Guðlaugur was present to hand out the results, to help publicize the need for self-deploying life rafts among the Icelandic fishing fleet.

Now I head over to the Vestmannaeyjar swimming hall, the one built after the lava flowed over the old pool. On this blustery, snowy morning, the island's famous winter winds are howling; some of the highest wind speeds in Europe have been recorded on the southern end of Heimaey. I learn something of Iceland's deep swimming culture from Guðlaugur's loquacious opposite, Alan Allison, who is now one of the two organizers in charge of Guðlaugssund. Alan has worked at the Vestmannaeyjar swimming hall for twenty years, as a lifeguard and pool manager.

Before arriving on Heimaey, I spent much of the previous week visiting public pools on the Icelandic mainland. What I came to understand from the experience is that even in winter—no, *especially* in winter—everybody is in the pool. Iceland is one of the world's leaders in swimming pools per capita. There's a special Icelandic road sign for it: a head poking out of two rows of blue waves. Most every town in the country, no matter how tiny, has a public pool—typically outdoors, often geothermally heated for year-round use—and many towns have several options of varying size and temperature. Because of Heimaey's unusually high winds, Vestmannaeyjar's offerings include an indoor lap pool. Every day, Alan tells me, the swimming hall sees multiple generations of Icelanders from all ages and backgrounds: the before-work swimmers, elementary schoolers during gym class, retirees coming for their recreation.

A few months before my arrival in Iceland, I'd read in the Icelandic newspapers about a group of thirty ocean swimmers preparing for a swim expedition in Reykjavík. Who should show up to join the swim but the president of Iceland, Guðni Jóhannesson? Local reporters observed that President Guðni shrugged off his unexpected appearance by welcoming the swimmers and declaring that "he doesn't doubt the health benefits of taking a dip in cold ocean water." At the end of the swim, the swimmers were invited to the presidential residence to warm themselves up in the president's own hot pool.

Alan says the ubiquitous hot pools throughout the country are what make Icelandic swimming special. After we do our laps inside the Vestmannaeyjar hall, we meander outdoors across the snow-covered ground so I can choose one of three hot pools in which to have a chat (temperature range: hot, very hot, extremely hot). Svenni Guðmundsson, the other organizer of Guðlaugssund, climbs down from his lifeguard station to join our conversation. He tells me that the pool will host "disco nights" for the local teenagers, during which he pipes popular music through the outdoor speakers. (At the moment, we are listening to the Rolling Stones, but "the teens don't know who the Rolling Stones are," he says, rolling his eyes.) The pool is how Icelanders survive the long, dark winter.

We discuss the evolution of Guðlaugssund, which started like this: On the first anniversary of the trawling accident, in March 1985, twenty students from the island's navigation college swam six kilometers in a pool, fully clothed, under the supervision of the then headmaster, Friðrik Ásmundsson, who had a reputation for strictness: no flotation devices, no holding on to the side of the pool. In those early years, the number of students participating in any given event went as high as seventy, but mostly held steady at two or three dozen, and the emphasis was on safety.

Beginning in 2000, the swim was opened to the public. High school students swam relays, local businesses sponsored their employees, and the island's swim team always had a healthy contingent. Fishing captains and other seamen were also well represented. Some swimmers asked to participate remotely, from nearby Reykjavík and as far away as Tibet and Vietnam. Almost everyone had an island or Icelandic connection.

Svenni's father is the captain of a fishing trawler, and he himself spent five winters on the sea. He tells me that he swims "for both the memory of Guðlaugur, who did this, and all the guys who didn't make it. We still think this swim is a reminder for everybody for safety, of equipment and also of swimming." He and Alan have swum numerous times, both individually and as part of the sports center's relay team.

Alan is unfailingly upbeat in his encouragement of first-time swimmers of all ages and abilities. The aim of the swim these days, he explains, is to have people achieve something they would not have thought they could accomplish themselves. Months before, over the course of my first phone conversation with Alan about Guðlaugssund, I somehow ended up agreeing to swim in it. "And if you can't finish the six kilometers," he cheerfully told me then, "I'll finish it for you."

Later at the swimming hall, I watch one young man stroll past the hot pools for a dip in the cold pool—the only outdoor pool that's unheated. The air temperature is twenty-six degrees, and there's ice on the ground. Forty-five-degree water is the kind of cold that is hard to imagine; to feel it for myself, I cautiously inch down the icy ramp, swearing under my breath at every step. What does it feel like? Piercing, and urgent. My cells scream for me to get out. Though I will later swim the full six kilometers of Guðlaugssund, it occurs to me that this plunge is probably the closest I'll ever come to feeling something of what Guðlaugur felt on his swim.

LIKE ANY GOOD Icelander, Guðlaugur often swam in the sea as a child. He and a friend would pinball from one side of the island to the other, swimming near the harbor, then near the lighthouse. It would take less than an hour for the pair of ten-year-olds to walk from town to a sweeping crescent-shaped black-sand beach on the south end of Heimaey. They thought nothing of it, until his friend's father got wind of it and put limits on their unsupervised ocean jaunts.

Guðlaugur and I are driving south past this very same crescent-shaped beach, toward the island's lighthouse, in his maroon Ford pickup truck. On the night of his swim, in the inky darkness and surging waves, the lighthouse is what guided him home. This evening, it's not quite dusk yet; the sun is low in the sky, bathing everything in a rose-gold tint, including Guðlaugur's big, silvery beard. I ask him if swimming still feels joyful to him. By way of an answer, he tells me about the time he and his wife went to the Westfjords region of Iceland, where they stayed at a place with a little infinity pool by the sea. Being in that pool, he says, was like being the sea itself. And it felt good.

We get out of his truck at the lighthouse and walk a little way over a field of parched, snow-covered grass. Installed on the cliff top is a waist-high circular memorial; on its surface is a weathered, coppery disc etched with a map of the island, with markings of our current location, the place where the boat went down, and the distance back to shore. The wind is wicked and sharp, whipping my hair into my face. Guðlaugur raises a hand and points southeast toward the sea.

"Much of the time, when something goes wrong on a fishing boat, everyone drowns," Guðlaugur says. "So there is no one to say what happened. But when we were holding on to the keel that night, we said that if one of us made it, we would tell them." He pauses. "I was there to tell." He faithfully kept his promise with the early decades of Guðlaugssund and with his vocal support for auto-deploying life rafts for all of Iceland's fishing fleet.

During my few days visiting the island, we go for several long drives, looping around on empty roads that trace the contours of the stark, red-rock landscape. The local population balloons in summer, when one-fifth of the world's puffins come back to roost on the Vestmannaeyjar archipelago, along with the thousands of human tourists who come to see them. In the winter months, though, tourism is largely dormant, and the island is returned to its year-round residents. In this small-town place, Guðlaugur explains, driving is the easiest way to have a conversation uninterrupted by someone he knows.

Guðlaugur is recognized everywhere in Iceland. "Well, you see, I don't blend in," he says wryly. At six-foot-four, he is a broad, striking man, with shoulder-length curly silver hair and a full beard edged with dark. If you Googled

"Hemingway" and "fisherman," you'd expect him, or someone who looks like him, to emerge in the search results. We
find out there is a French film crew in the area, out on a boat,
making a documentary about him. Guðlaugur doesn't speak
with them, but he knows they're there. He gets phone calls
from journalists in Japan. When he visits his children and
grandchildren in Reykjavík, people often come up to him in
public to shake his hand and to ask how his life has been.

On one evening drive, we see the lights of two cod-fishing
vessels returning to the harbor. I insist that we stop at a fish
restaurant so he can let me buy him dinner. On our way out,
a smiling woman with smartly cut hair and stylish black
boots approaches, and I assume it's another admirer. "My
sister," he says shyly, introducing us.

What I learn is that he lives on the same street where he
grew up; his wife, Maria, grew up on that street, too. They live
in the house where she was born. One morning, they invite
me over for brunch, and Maria shows me the vegetable plots
in their tidy backyard garden. Behind the garden, Guðlaugur
builds things, like a tall wood stove fashioned from part of a
fishing trawler. He is busy with work, family, friends, travels.
Once, in the year after his accident, he swam in Lake George,
in upstate New York, the lake my husband and I swam across
the morning after we were married. Somehow, learning this
makes us feel like kin to one another.

On one wall of his home, in a place of honor, there is
a framed piece of art made by his grandson, Daniel, when
Daniel was in kindergarten. It's a brightly colored sand

painting of a blue-ocean background, a red fishing boat, and, next to it, the dark figure of a man swimming in the water. When Guðlaugur and Maria show this picture to me, I am surprised by the tears that suddenly prick my eyes.

WHAT CAN GUÐLAUGUR *tell us?* is the question at hand. But perhaps the more important corollary is, *Will Guðlaugur tell us what we want to know?* I began to realize that the stories other swimmers told about Guðlaugur were just as revealing about human nature as anything the man himself could tell me. And I came to understand that I had to visit Heimaey to witness both kinds of stories for myself.

Alan Allison introduces me to Sigrún Halldórsdóttir, a young teacher who moved from Vestmannaeyjar to Reykjavík and is now a swim coach. Three years ago, she began to lead her charges in swimming Guðlaugssund. Sigrún started swimming Guðlaugssund when she was twelve years old. She is now thirty. "Even after I stopped swim team, I do the swim every year on my own, to keep it alive," Sigrún tells me when I phone her up. "It's a big deal, what he did." She teaches her swim team about Guðlaugur's achievement; after the children complete their swims, Alan mails them signed certificates from Vestmannaeyjar. Hearing from them illuminates the Everyman side of this saga: Guðlaugur's story tells us that we swim for survival, but also that we swim for remembrance.

After the accident, from his hospital bed, Guðlaugur spoke with a television interviewer about his experience. In the footage, his face is young, cherubic. He wears a faint wispy mustache and a white hospital gown. His eyes downcast, he talks about the seagulls, who circled above his head as he swam. He spoke to them and asked them to get help if they could. All night long, they stayed above him.

The Icelandic doctor who conducted the medical studies became a good friend. A few years ago, they met each other over coffee. The doctor told Guðlaugur that he'd just been to a medical conference on hypothermia. Many of the other doctors had the same question about his most famous patient. "Is he all right in the head?" they asked. When people go through something so big, they can go crazy. Guðlaugur told the doctor that he was fine; he joked that he couldn't get any crazier than he already was.

Guðlaugur explains to me that during his recovery, his father sat in a chair next to his bed at the hospital and didn't leave his side for a month. Guðlaugur felt compelled to talk. He would relay the drama of the accident over and over again, and his father would listen. "I think that is why I am OK now," he tells me. "My father was a very good listener." It's his father's startlingly beautiful cursive handwriting that fills the pages of the Guðlaugssund logbook, recounting the events of that night with care and recording the swims and their participants, year after year, for posterity.

At the Vestmannaeyjar history museum, the clothes Guðlaugur wore the night of his swim are hanging in a glass case. His mother saved them and carefully put them away; eventually, his wife donated them to the museum.

"We all want to survive. We all have a will to do it," says Helga Hallbergsdóttir, the director of the museum, and a friend of Guðlaugur's. "But I think that conversation at the top of the boat, before it sank, they promised one another—that if someone somehow survives, that he will work to make things safer and better, to save others—that's what kept him going."

Guðlaugur didn't choose to swim for his life. But if there's meaning in what happened, perhaps it is that his survival, enabled by swimming, encouraged others to learn to swim, too. I ask Helga why she thinks the islanders still swim Guðlaugssund so faithfully, year in and year out, nearly thirty-five years later. She says that his accomplishment is a reminder of all those who did not survive, and of our own inevitable mortality. "We have not forgotten what he was able to do," she says, "and we respect him very much for it." The emphasis on swimming instruction that began on this island, by extension, is now baked into the cultural DNA of Iceland itself.

"The pool," Helga tells me with a smile, "is our pub."

After all these years, and after all his reservations, why did Guðlaugur agree to talk to me? It becomes clear, in the few days we spend together, that it was because the cultural DNA that lives in his fellow Icelanders lives in him, too.

He makes it a point to tell me this story: Three weeks before, he'd gone to the hardware store in town. On his way in from the parking lot, he ran into someone he knew, a woman who would be turning ninety years old that weekend. He bid her a good day. She looked up at him without recognition: *Do we know each other?* "I said, 'Don't you remember me?'" She was his swimming teacher, the one who taught him how to swim in the old swimming pool, fifty years before. He doesn't often go out of his way to remind people who he is, but he wanted her to remember that she'd taught him to swim. "I said, 'Well, it turned out well for me.'" He pauses and smiles. "And then she understood who I was."

I WAKE EARLY in the morning for Guðlaugssund. There's fresh snow on the ground, and I crunch through it on my walk to the pool in the six a.m. gloom.

Five swimmers, four men and one woman, are already in the water, having braved the predawn cold at four-thirty a.m. so that they could complete the swim and still get to work on time. Alan and Svenni are manning the officials' table; they introduce me to the partners and friends and coworkers sitting on the pool deck. Some are counting laps. Some are there to keep company. More swimmers show up, ready to go. Under my bare feet, the red tile floor is clammy and damp. As I wait for a lane to open up, I think about how everyone is here for the same thing.

The routine tradition of it is reminiscent of Thanksgiving Day turkey trots and Fourth of July fun runs. On a Wednesday morning in the second week of March, in this small-town Icelandic pool, we are paying homage to a man, and to a country's history, through a national pastime. It's not quite a national holiday. Instead of hot dogs and fireworks, there's hot coffee and two hundred and forty laps. In a modest, mundane way, this is simply how a community binds itself together. But in the doggedness, there is something bigger and more beautiful than the thirty people in the swimming hall.

When I do get in the water, I find that the swim is something that largely takes place inside my head. I settle in, and eventually I notice things. At two kilometers, I watch the elementary school headmaster in the next lane haul himself out and head off to work. At three kilometers, I smell fish, when Svenni opens the outside door. The fishmeal factory is up and running for the day. At four kilometers, the sun has risen enough so that it starts to filter through the skylights and side windows, a glorious late-winter lemon yellow. It plays across the lanes and down into the water where I swim.

At five kilometers, I start feeling giddy. I am reminded of the warning posted by the hot pools: *Caution! Excessive use of hot tubs may cause dysphoria.* With eight laps to go, I poke my head up and do the breaststroke, double-checking my distance with Alan, who's counting my laps. I finish with one lap each of butterfly, backstroke, breaststroke, and freestyle, just to mix it up, just to show I am still in good form. An hour and fifty minutes after I begin, I'm done. I text Guðlaugur to let him know that I have completed the swim in his honor. It gives me great pleasure to be able to do this. He calls from work to caution me, in an avuncular way, to make sure I get some rest. It is a long swim, after all, he says. I think about how surreal it is that he's the one telling me that. Then I walk back through the snow to my hotel and take a nap.

VISITING THE ICELANDIC coast, contemplating the sea from the perch of a pool: it is swimming as liturgy. The rite of swimming enables us to endure many things through a communal call-and-response of story as well as practice. I believe in the power of how we pass down that tradition.

In many ways, swimming and family were intertwined for me from the start. It's my own origin story. In the summer of 1968, my parents met in a swimming pool in Hong Kong. For one hot moment, they were the cliché incarnate: he was the bronzed lifeguard, she was the bikini-clad beauty with long black hair and big, serious eyes. When I flip through snapshots of that time, I can hardly bear their prettiness: their slim-limbed stances, the way they looked at each other with such longing.

Such longing, of course, rarely lasts. That they stayed married as many years as they did—until my older brother and I were safely in college—is complicated by periods of living apart, blowout fights, silent treatments. The only things they had in common, it seemed, were their youthful looks, us kids, and swimming.

People who know my brother and me laugh when we tell them our parents met at the pool. We began to swim at ages six and five at the outdoor recreation center near our home on Long Island. As the precursor to a life in the water—the final mileage not yet marked—I spent summer mornings taking lessons with Andy while our mother swam laps in the next lane. Her favorite stroke was breaststroke. As we paddled alongside, we could see her head popping up for breath at regular intervals, her legs executing a powerful frog kick under the calm surface.

In the afternoons, my father would sometimes join us, and we'd head down to Jones Beach. We drove the eight miles along the causeway from our house, leapfrogging across the little islands in the bay that separate fish-shape Long Island from the skinny barrier island that is the beach. On the other side of that barrier island was the vast viridian-green expanse of the Atlantic Ocean. We rolled down the windows and let the sea air blast through our eggshell-colored 1978 Volvo station wagon; during low tide, we pinched our noses against the stink that rose from the exposed mudflats below.

Most visits my mother and father would begin with a jog alone together by the water's edge. At the end of the run they'd jump into the ocean, and my father would finish with a solo swim beyond the shore break. This was his comfort zone: Every stroke pulled him further from us, back in time to the days spent free diving and spearfishing with his father and brother off the subtropical beaches of Hong Kong Island. My mother would come back and sit on the towel, and we'd look up every now and again, shading our eyes, searching out my father's splashing figure in the waves. Swimming out there was a grown-up thing. Each year I hopefully inched closer and closer to it.

My parents seemed so happy in the water. In real life, on land, they were often at odds. She was the stern, responsible parent who ran the household and paid the bills. He got to be the fun one, the artist who worked in his downstairs studio and stayed up until four a.m. They never talked about the things that mattered: why he felt lonely in America or what she missed of life outside of raising kids. It was a wonder they agreed on swimming. But at those moments on the beach, or in the pool with us, I believed they still loved each other. In the water, the rigid roles that were so defined at home disappeared. The allure of swimming, already powerful, was amplified by its association with the tenuous thing that still held my parents together.

We were a family, and then we weren't. No one in our foursome kept swimming except for me. I swam through the divorce. I swam through college. I swam from Alcatraz, on a dare. I swam as rehab from knee surgery. I swam across a lake at my wedding. I swam to an Italian monastery and back, to help settle someone else's bet. I swam through a miscarriage and on each of the days before my two sons were born. Three decades of swimming, of chasing equilibrium, have kept my head firmly above water. Swimming can enable survival in ways beyond the physical.

Survival stories like those of Guðlaugur and ancient swimmers like the Moken have to do with me as a swimmer, too. Reading the Australian philosopher Damon Young helps me to understand the importance of the sublime in our experience of swimming. Eighteenth-century philosophers explained the sublime and its power in the meeting of nature's opposing forces and ideas: pain and pleasure, terror and awe, fear and exhilaration, life and death. When we swim today, writes Young, that euphoria "comes from the passions of survival, without the desperate need *to* survive." We come closer to the acutely vivid experience of life itself.

We evolve. Why we swim does, too.

WELL-BEING

~

How nice it would be to die swimming toward the sun.

—LE CORBUSIER

One of the best marathon swimmers in the world today began swimming as an adult, in 2009, to rehab a leg she almost lost to amputation. A high-heel shoe was the culprit, Kim Chambers tells me—it led to a nasty fall down the stairs outside her San Francisco apartment. She remembers the doctors telling her this: *We saved your leg, but we don't know what—if any—functionality you'll ever have.* It took her two years to learn how to walk again. It took much less time to discover that she is freakishly gifted at long-distance swimming.

You could say that Kim is the best swimmer in the world whom you don't know. Seven months after she first got into a pool after her accident, she swam from Alcatraz to San Francisco, cutting across the choppy waters and fierce currents of San Francisco Bay. She now holds multiple world records for distance swimming, including one she set in 2015 by becoming the first woman to swim solo from the Farallon Islands to the Golden Gate Bridge, a thirty-mile journey that began with her slipping into pitch-dark waters just before midnight in the notorious Red Triangle of great white sharks. It took her just over seventeen hours; under the watchful eye of her boat crew, she faced nausea, high winds, and the perpetual menace of sharks. Ever thoughtful, Kim did her laundry and folded it neatly the night before; she didn't want to leave a mess in case she didn't make it back. She was only the sixth person in history to complete the Oceans Seven, the open-water swimming equivalent of the Seven Summits. This consists of the English Channel, the Strait of Gibraltar, the Molokai Channel, Lake Tahoe, the Cook Strait in New Zealand, the Tsugaru Strait in Japan, and the North Channel from Ireland to Scotland, after which she went into toxic shock from hundreds of jellyfish stings.

One gray, drizzly December morning, I join Kim for a swim in San Francisco Bay. I want to get a sense of the way that swimming is a daily practice for her, and how it got that way. The water temperature is a brisk fifty-three degrees Fahrenheit, the air forty-eight. "The days I don't get in are the days I don't feel right," she tells me as we contemplate the bay from Aquatic Park, the sandy beach behind the Dolphin Club, one of the premier open-water swimming and rowing clubs in the world. It was founded in 1877. Its neighbor, the South End Rowing Club, is even older; it was founded in 1873. Both are institutions, with numerous Olympians on their century-and-a-half-old membership rolls. They are fierce yet friendly rivals, and Kim is a member of both clubs. "I'm a middle child," she says sheepishly, by way of explanation.

For many swimmers, the act of swimming is a tonic, in

that old-fashioned sense of the word: it is a restorative, a stimulant, undertaken for a feeling of vigor and well-being. The word *tonic* comes from the Greek *tonikos*, "of or for stretching." About a dozen people are in the water already, swimming against the unlikely backdrop of ships and industrial docks and tall-masted sailboats. Rain pocks the steely surface of the water, a liquid-mercury mirror of the sky above. There is an expansiveness here. It's not too hard to think of this kind of swimming as stretching the mind as well as the body.

Kim stops to greet Stella, the sopping-wet dog of a fellow Dolphin Club member. The dog yelps and jumps, licking Kim's face and hands in excitement. Me, I can't stop shivering, even in a four-millimeter neoprene wetsuit. Kim is unfazed. Five-feet-ten and willowy, with a high-megawatt smile, she shakes out her arms but otherwise shows no signs of cold—only a puppyish eagerness to get in the water. Others here are of a similar mind. Eighty-year-old Mimi, who swims from the club every morning, grins at us as she strides purposefully down the wood-planked stairs to the water. Like Kim, she is outfitted simply in a cap, goggles, and a thin one-piece Lycra swimsuit. Wetsuits aren't exactly frowned upon here—the club encourages all comers—but swimmers are gently encouraged to do without.

It still amazes Kim that she just happened to stumble into one of the best training grounds there is for what she does. At the time she began swimming with the club, though, she was just trying to survive. The treatment for her leg injury—a blunt force trauma that caused a catastrophic buildup of pressure inside one of her leg compartments—required multiple surgeries to relieve pressure, as well as skin grafts, hyperbaric treatments, and a stint in the burn unit at San Francisco's St. Francis Hospital. Two years later, she finally went back to work. "I was most worried about the scars," she tells me. "My gait was off. I couldn't go for a run. And I didn't feel like me." She hid her scars under long pants and wore dark shoes to camouflage the clunky orthotics she needed to support her stride.

She remembered the freedom of being in the water as a child in New Zealand, so she worked up the courage to begin swimming at a local pool—in the evenings, because she didn't want people ogling her scars. Her first goal was to swim a mile. At first, her stroke was terrible. Kim's mentor, the entrepreneur and investor Vito Bialla, an accomplished open-water swimmer in his own right, would later say that when he first met her she couldn't swim her way out of a paper bag with flippers on. One day, two swimmers in the pool asked her if she'd ever thought about swimming in the bay. *Swimming in the bay?* she wondered. Kim had been living in San Francisco since 1995, but she'd never heard of anyone swimming in the bay.

On a crisp fifty-four-degree day in Aquatic Park, in late 2009, Kim gave it a try. Despite the cold, she couldn't stop smiling the whole time. She joined the Dolphin Club the next month. She calls it a secret society of adventurers, populated by individuals of all ages and incomes. Sometimes it takes a while for her to recognize a fellow member on the street: "It's because they're wearing clothes for a change," she says. When Kim and I first meet, she is on the verge of turning forty; these days she has no qualms about talking about her scars. She shows me her right leg, neat tracks circumscribing the skin graft that was taken from her upper thigh to repair the traumatized tissue around her calf. "The water has been my teacher. It is my sanctuary. You can have a shitty week, but then you come to the water and feel cleansed. You're naked— all the artifice is stripped away." I begin to understand that the scars are a map of how she rehabilitated her life.

The morning of our first swim together, Kim claps her hands and hoots, the wordless sound a kind of blessing. "Ready?" she asks. We dive in and stroke our way toward Alcatraz.

5

The Water Cure

While posted in London in the 1750s, Benjamin Franklin swam daily in the Thames. The cold bath was a corrective much in vogue, and the scientist, inventor, and all-around Renaissance man was an avid skinny-dipper for much of his long life. Brits at the time suffered from what one writer has called "a mess of maladies . . . fevers, digestive complaints, melancholia, nervous tics, tremors, and even stupidity were the epidemics of the day." The new wonder drug prescribed for the nasty health effects of urban living? Cold seawater. And thus the English seaside resort was born—not for sun worshipping or frolicking, but for dunking oneself in the cold miracle cure of the ocean. It was the collective baptism of a country.

Back across the pond, water therapy became big business in nineteenth-century America. Public distrust of the medical establishment led to the fervent adoption of the water cure for everything from broken bones to typhus. There was even a hydropathic medical school, opened in New York City in 1851. By the outbreak of the Civil War, more than two hundred water cure clinics were operating around the country, and a journal dedicated to the subject had tens of thousands of subscribers.

"Water cure patients sat in water, submerged themselves in water, stood under water as it was poured over them, wore wet compresses, wrapped themselves in dripping sheets, and ate a meager diet washed down, of course, with water," writes one historian of the practices. It was water, water everywhere—mostly for immersion but sometimes to drink. (The prescription of eight glasses of water a day is a relic from this time.) Cold water was proclaimed the sovereign remedy for every ailment. Dunk your head in it for a fever! Sniff it for a nosebleed! Take a cold mouth-bath to cure yourself of the filthy habit of tobacco chewing and restore a healthy salivary flow!

Swimming was critical to the water cure. In the eight-volume *Hydropathic Encyclopedia*, published circa 1851, the "swimming-bath" is prescribed as "health preserving" and "hygienic" for all persons, but also as "eminently therapeutic in some forms of chronic disease." As I flip through the encyclopedia's five hundred plus pages, I find its exhaustive discussions of river, sponge, and wave baths to be both mind-numbing and fascinating. Whether you were weak in the lungs from tuberculosis or suffering from chronic constipation, swimming would help—to strengthen and open up the lungs, to get those lax abdominal muscles going and (ahem) move things along. Pamphlets rained down on the public prescribing saltwater swims for longevity.

Our trust in water as a cure-all goes back to the ancients. Egyptian royals bathed in water laced with essential oils, and Chinese and Japanese traditions extolled the medicinal effects of thermal springs. The Greeks went deep in their examination of every type of water therapy. Euripides wrote that "the sea restores men's health"—with great personal gratitude, since he was allegedly cured of rabies with a near drowning in the ocean. Called the "sailors' method," this combination of water and asphyxia was a celebrated ancient treatment for the disease. One symptom of rabies is hydrophobia, and it was thought that a timely application of water would cure it. (Euripides notwithstanding, it did not prove to be an effective remedy.) Hippocrates and Aristotle were big fans of hot seawater baths. Romans would soak in hot water pools, then hop into the frigidarium—a bracing cold-water bath—to close the pores and leave bathers refreshed at the end of the regimen.

For most of this history of immersing our bodies in water for wellness, proponents didn't know exactly what they were talking about when it came to why. But they knew what felt good.

KIM CHAMBERS DOESN'T know much about the murky history of the water cure, but she was desperate to recover after her injury. When she fell that day in 2007, she smacked her head on the ground and struck her leg on a big ceramic pot at the bottom of the stairs. "I have a really high pain tolerance," she tells me, "so I just thought it was going to be a nasty bruise." She managed to drive to work, her leg ballooning to nearly double its normal size. At the office, she collapsed. At the hospital, surgeons sliced open her leg in two places to relieve the swelling that was destroying her nerves. She didn't wake up until postsurgery, when her doctors reported the grim news that she might never walk again.

What does despair look like, feel like? It looks like angry red scars. It feels like shame, the urgent desire to hide a limp. It feels like desperation. It is the opposite, then, of the unfettered joy of a child swimming at the beach.

That joy is what Kim was after when she made herself go to the pool. Being a patient gets old after a while—two years of doctors' appointments, pain meds, full-time physical therapy. On the morning she swam for the first time in San Francisco Bay, what she finally found was a glimpse of an alternate reality. "Not a lot of people have video footage of their rebirth," Kim says. "But I do. The guys I was swimming with filmed me, this shivering, skinny, broken woman who was a hundred and twenty pounds soaking wet. But I had the biggest shit-eating grin on my face that they'd ever seen." It occurs to me that religious people who find God, of course, do have videos of their rebirth. They are born again—oftentimes in water, with a baptism.

After Kim started swimming in the cold waters of the bay, she noticed a change in her severely nerve-damaged right leg: it had more feeling in it. She had a theory that she ran by her physicians in those early days. "All the blood is sucked from your extremities to protect your organs when you get in that cold water," she explains, in her lilting New Zealand accent, during one of our marathon phone calls after work one evening. (When she's not training or traveling the world for swims, she has until recently been working as a director of community engagement for Adobe, the software company.) "Couldn't it be possible that when the blood rushes back into those extremities after you warm up again, that you're getting a kind of oxygen therapy? That there's a higher rate of it being flushed around your body?" Her doctors said they could see the validity in it, with oxygen circulating at a much faster rate than if Kim were sedentary or even exercising on land. The result: her nerves were regenerating at a swifter pace relative to that of the previous two years.

TO TEASE APART the tangle of truth and myth around water, I call up Dr. Hirofumi Tanaka, director of the Cardiovascular Aging Research Laboratory and professor of kinesiology at the University of Texas. He studies how our bodies move, heal, and age. By virtue of his work, and his upbringing—in the string of islands that is Japan, where learning to swim is required of all schoolchildren—Tanaka is an effusive, enthusiastic proponent of swimming for health.

Tanaka's lab has pioneered new research on swimming's effects on two of the biggest hallmarks of aging: high blood pressure and arthritis. "Over the last four or five years, a funky thing happened—we realized that the effects of swimming actually surpassed the magnitude of the effects of walking or cycling," he tells me. "None of us knew that before." Average reduction in blood pressure after land-based exercise training is five to seven points. Swimming, he found, reduces blood pressure by an average of nine points—in the blood-pressure world, that's significant. It also decreases arterial stiffness, a condition in which the walls of your arteries become less elastic and add strain to the heart muscle.

The pressure of water itself on your body plays a part in swimming for health. When you immerse yourself in water, it pushes blood away from the extremities and toward your heart and lungs; this temporarily elevates your blood pressure and makes your heart and lungs work harder. The process builds efficiency and endurance in the cardiovascular system, leading to lower blood pressure over time. And when you swim, the water provides gentle, all-around resistance for your muscles to work against.

There's an element of agelessness to swimming, Tanaka says: more bodies can do this, and for longer. In Japan, a nation of old people, swimming is hugely popular. There is even a subset of Japanese manga, or comic books, dedicated to swimming. Tanaka loves to go up to the top of Tokyo Skytree—at two thousand and eighty feet, it's the tallest tower in the world—because on a clear day you can look down and see all the swimming pools glinting on the city's rooftops.

Swimming had always been assumed to be good treatment for arthritis, but there was no science to back it up. In 2016, Tanaka and his co-researchers published a paper that provided a definitive *yes*. "If you look at patients with arthritis, the major issues are pain and function," Tanaka says. "They suffer from chronic pain on a daily basis. After swimming training, the pain levels went down substantially. And even though the patients were in water, the functions we assessed on land—walking, standing from a chair—improved substantially. Swimming is the best exercise we can prescribe because it stimulates mobility—without pain—and circulation." The swimming studies were done in cool water pools, that is, regular swimming pools, which are typically eighty degrees and below.

So Kim Chambers's instinct was right: swimming in cool water every day boosted her vascular function—the healthy circulation of blood around the body, to the damaged parts that needed it—even more than running or cycling would have. And, perhaps most important, without the pain.

"If I don't swim, the pain grows. If I'm in more pain, what will become of my life?" In an essay on living with chronic pain, the writer Melissa Hung describes a swim as a daily act of endurance. In the years since a headache has taken up permanent residence inside her skull, the pool is the place where pain leaves center stage, if only briefly. It's where she finds momentary relief from "a body that will not behave." Swimming hurts, but not swimming hurts more.

President Franklin D. Roosevelt suffered from polio; while in office, he had a swimming pool installed in the White House and swam for therapy several times a day. President John F. Kennedy, who endured near-constant back pain and a life of excruciating health miseries, loved the pool so much he swam before lunch and dinner. FDR's pool remains there today, beneath what is the press pool briefing room.

Buoyancy, floating, weightlessness. Freedom. These are the words we use to talk about swimming. Is it a coincidence that this is also the language we use to talk about the lightness of being, the wellness of being, that we strive for in this corporeal world?

Downstairs at the Dolphin Club, between the boathouse and the front stairway entrance, there's a quote from Henry David Thoreau's *Walden* posted on the wall: "Renew thyself completely each day; do it again, & again, & forever again."

"You do renew yourself every time you're out there," Kim tells me one day, as we look out at the bay from the upstairs window of the boathouse. Over the course of the winter and spring, we continue to meet up periodically for swims. On this particular morning, it's proving to be a stormy start, and the water is turbulent. "We all have bad days and heartache and heartbreak. But you submerge yourself in that water, and it's like pressing the reset button. It has given me tremendous clarity." Each time she gets in, it's as if the water reflects how she feels and responds in kind. "That's why I have to do it every day."

Swimming from the Farallon Islands, thirty miles out in the Pacific, was for Kim the ultimate extension of how being in deep water could force a kind of surrender. As she likes to put it, the five-mile radius around the islands is the great white sharks' living room. She's just a visitor, passing through. After her record-breaking swims as part of the first all-female relay team from the Farallons and then as the first solo woman, despite the danger, she would swim there every day if she could. She sometimes takes a weekend jaunt out to the islands, just to swim.

"All my senses are ignited," she says. "I can smell the sea life. That feeling of being in water that's six thousand or ten thousand feet deep, and you're just this tiny person swimming on the surface." Entrepreneur Vito Bialla has described swimming at the Farallons as akin to being in heaven and talking to the devil at the same time. The restlessness of the seascape, Kim says, is captivating for her. "You don't know what's swimming underneath you. The seals all around, and the birds. You know you're not supposed to be there, and a shark could come out of nowhere. It's tantalizing to be on that edge, to be that connected."

Before her accident, Kim was a self-described control freak—about her body, about her appearance, about her weight. She had a job in Silicon Valley with long hours and good money. "I was a superficial person," she says. "I was classically trained as a ballerina, and everything in my world view was very disciplined." Learning to swim meant learning how to relinquish control, to thrive in a space of uncertainty.

She works hard to prepare for each big swim, but she now finds nothing more exhilarating than jumping in and not knowing what will come. "We live a life on land, and we think we know what's going to happen," she tells me, "but we don't. And I've learned how to surrender. It's so freeing, and so scary, but you feel like this modern-day explorer. Not many people have gotten into the water in the Farallons. You're like an astronaut out there." In 2016, Kim was inducted into the Explorers Club, which includes among its members astronauts and explorers, including Sir Edmund Hillary, Tenzing Norgay, Sylvia Earle, Neil Armstrong, Sally Ride, Thor Heyerdahl, and Jane Goodall.

During the course of our morning swims, I learn from Kim that the daily swim in the bay is where she confronts her demons. Then she shakes their hands. Ten years ago, she was someone who wasn't supposed to walk again. And yet here she is, a multiple world-record holder in a discipline that, back then, she didn't even know existed. It's human nature to resist doing things that are uncomfortable for us. But she finds something extraordinary in pushing through the discomfort to see what's on the other side.

ONE FALL, I decided to swim from Alcatraz to San Francisco. I did it on a dare. What I remember most about a nighttime tour I once took of the island prison is the fact that, given the nearness of Alcatraz to downtown San Francisco, inmates were often haunted by the sounds of life across the water. When city residents held New Year's Eve parties and their reveling carried across the cold, current-roiled bay, the shore seemed maddeningly close to the prisoners. It was the ultimate torture—that of proximity.

Alcatraz's barren, craggy island is less than a square mile in area. Everywhere there are astounding views of San

Francisco, the expansive bay, and the rust-hued Golden Gate Bridge. Ohlone oral history tells us that Alcatraz was used by the indigenous people as a place of isolation, to punish those who violated tribal law. When you are there, especially at night, you understand. It makes sense that you would feel small anchored in a place so big.

In the nearly three decades that Alcatraz, known as the Rock, was a functioning federal prison—from 1934 to 1963, when it closed due to the skyrocketing costs of having to bring in everything by boat, including fresh water—it held high-risk prisoners, including Al Capone, Robert Stroud (aka the Birdman of Alcatraz, so called because he became a respected ornithologist during his earlier incarceration at Leavenworth penitentiary), and Roy Gardner, the great American train robber and the most notorious escape artist of his time. Transferred to Alcatraz in 1934, Gardner successfully appealed for clemency and was released in July 1938; the next year, he published a sensational autobiography. He named the book after the place that marked him: *Hellcatraz*. In another year, he would be dead, by suicide.

The Rock is a place that can drive you mad. As a prison, it had a storied menace. It was designed to break you into submission. All in all, there were fourteen separate documented escape attempts involving thirty-six prisoners. Of these, the most infamous and exhaustively planned attempt was that of Frank Morris and the Anglin brothers, in June 1962. They tunneled out of their cells using sharpened spoons; in their beds they left blankets and dummy heads constructed out of soap, toilet paper, and their own hair. In the dead of night, they entered the water in an inflated raft made from fifty stolen raincoats. The three men were never found, but a recent study using computer modeling and historical tide information from that date shows a very narrow window of opportunity in which they could have avoided being sucked out to sea. It is possible that they were able to get out of the water in the headlands north of the Golden Gate Bridge—debris from this landing would likely have washed up on Angel Island after the tide turned—and this in fact was where the FBI found a paddle and personal items linked to the men. Still, the most probable outcome was hypothermia, and drowning.

One inmate, John Paul Scott, succeeded in swimming from the island to Fort Point, on the southern end of the Golden Gate Bridge, in December 1962. Scott's was the only confirmed case of a prisoner reaching the shore by swimming. The water temperature (typically below sixty degrees), vicious currents (often moving at six knots or faster), sharp-edged rocks (that could slice you to ribbons), and sharks (enough said) were believed to make the task futile. Scott proved it wasn't.

He and another prisoner had fashioned water wings from stolen rubber gloves (the two worked on kitchen duty; Scott's co-conspirator broke his ankle during the prison break and was captured within minutes). Scott ended up beached at Fort Point during an ebb tide and was found unconscious, suffering from hypothermia, by four teenagers. After a brief stay at the Presidio hospital, he was taken back to Alcatraz.

Surely it says something about our collective beliefs that we chose to put a maximum-security federal prison on a speck of land barely a mile and a half offshore from San Francisco. We build jails like Riker's Island—sandwiched between the Bronx and Queens and within shouting distance of the runways at New York's LaGuardia Airport—and prisons like Alcatraz tantalizingly close to our cities, and we believe them to be secure because of the water surrounding them.

But swimmers on the outside had been testing the waters around Alcatraz since at least the 1920s. Prior to its conversion to a federal prison, Alcatraz was used by the military both as a fortification and as a detention center (Confederate POWs were housed there early in the American Civil War). In 1933, the year before Alcatraz opened as a federal penitentiary, seventeen-year-old Anastasia Scott (no relation to the prisoner John Paul), whose father was a sergeant stationed on the island, swam from Alcatraz to San Francisco in forty-three minutes, accompanied by a rowboat. She was the first woman on record to make the swim. Two other San Francisco swimmers, Doris McLeod and Gloria Scigliano, followed shortly thereafter, to protest the decision to turn the island into a federal prison. McLeod completed a two-way crossing in two hours. All three women were excellent swimmers with knowledge of the tide conditions; also critical to their success, of course, was the fact that they were not required to escape under cover of darkness or to subsist on a prison diet with little to no exercise.

For our swim from the Rock, my friend Steve and I took up training in the waters around Aquatic Park, the end point for most Alcatraz swims; from this spot you can venture into the open bay and get a feel for the strength of the currents. The first time we swam there, I experienced a queasy discomfort—it started with a tightness in my chest and a genuine anxiety of the kind I had not felt for years when it came to swimming. My breath did not come easy. I did not know if I should attribute that to the cold, which felt unexpectedly crushing, or to the wetsuit, which felt unexpectedly confining. Steve smiled widely at me when we took a break to tread water and check in with each other. *Relax*, he said when he saw my face. *And breathe.*

By the morning of the swim itself, I had tried to prepare myself for the cold, and I was familiar with the way the bay's currents pull you with unnerving speed toward the open ocean on an outgoing tide. I knew that container ships could seem far away but come upon you in a matter of seconds. Our boat pilot, Gary Emich, was an open-water swimming legend who would go on to break a world record with his one-thousandth swim from Alcatraz to San Francisco. I had conditioned myself to follow Steve's advice: *Relax, and breathe.*

There were six of us swimming that day. The water temperature was fifty-seven degrees, the surface chopped with a light wind. We arrived at Alcatraz before nine a.m. and jumped in on a flood tide. The chilly water had a bite that managed to steal my first breath away. We regrouped for one last wave at our boat and its pilot. In photos from that morning, I am smiling. I look warmer than I felt, the sun glinting silver on my reflective goggles. We turned for the city and swam.

As I stroked through the water, I fell into a rhythm, and suddenly the swim didn't feel like a fight. There was an ease, a comforting regularity, to each round of breath, stroke, stroke, breath. We were prepared for it. The tight band that squeezed my chest upon entry loosened, and I began to greet the periodic cresting wave with aplomb instead of anxiety, skirting each rise of foam with an enthusiastic and carefully timed frog kick.

Other than the occasional rogue seaweed tangle, we managed to avoid any undesirable or hazardous run-ins with marine life. (Alas, sea lion bites have recently become a thing there.) The unusual fish-eye angle to the Golden Gate Bridge, and to Alcatraz, were reminders of the rarefied club in which we were earning membership. The forty-five minutes passed swiftly, and suddenly we arrived at Aquatic Park. Emich proclaimed it an excellent time.

6

Seawater in Our Veins

Get in the ocean every day, and your body will calibrate itself to the medium's moods, rhythms, temperatures. At fifty-three degrees, you get the ice cream headache. At fifty degrees, the bones in your wrists ache. On any given day, Kim and her fellow Dolphin Clubbers and South Enders can call the water temperature to within a degree, just by feel. "What'd you think it was today? Fifty-nine?" she wonders aloud to me in the water one day. When I ask why she thinks so, she says it's because it feels *wonderful*. "Yeah, I would bet a lot of money on that. It's not quite sixty . . . Let's swim over and check the thermometer." (She's right, of course.)

Human fetuses inhale and exhale amniotic fluid in utero, helping to form the lungs. We have so-called gill slits that become parts of our jaws and respiratory tracts, the form of which are evolutionary relics of aquatic, gill-breathing vertebrates. Seawater is so similar in mineral content to human blood plasma that our white blood cells can survive and function in it for some time. I delight in my mental picture of this, the not-so-fanciful notion that we have seawater circulating in our veins.

Since Guðlaugur's involuntary plunge into the sea more than three decades ago, science has been introduced to other humans with unusual adaptive abilities in extremely cold water. There's Lynne Cox, the legendary open-water swimmer who was the first to swim the Bering Strait; she swam from Alaska to the Soviet Union in 1987 in water that dropped as low as thirty-eight degrees. (The headline in the *New York Times* read LONG, COLD SWIM. Her reception was reported thusly: "It was a simple seaside picnic, a genteel tea party on the beach, but to get there took some doing for the guest of honor.") The following year, Guðlaugur and Cox appeared in the same academic journal, in a scholarly brief about the potential for Arctic swims to become a sport.

In 2002, Cox swam more than a mile in thirty-two-degree water in Antarctica—she was the first person ever to do so. In 2007, she swam in Disko Bay, Greenland, in water that was below twenty-seven degrees. The average American woman has a body fat percentage that ranges between 22 and 25 percent. Cox's body fat has been estimated at 35 percent; more significantly, it is very evenly distributed around her body. In addition to keeping her warm, this "internal wetsuit" provides her with neutral buoyancy in seawater, which means she can expend very little energy to maintain optimal swimming position in the ocean. Like Guðlaugur, Cox has participated in medical studies, opening researchers' eyes to new ways to treat multiple sclerosis (cold water swimming can dramatically reduce spasticity for a number of hours following immersion) and to improve hospital procedures around heart, spinal, and brain injuries (cooling the body can reduce swelling and trauma).

By studying the specifics of blood flow into Cox's hand while it was immersed in cold water, for example, doctors learned how to better plan for surgeries. Scientists also found that with immersion in cold water, Cox's core body temperature actually goes *up*. See what she can do when she enters a cold-water Jacuzzi: in two minutes, her body heat warms the water by two degrees Fahrenheit. (Guðlaugur has not undergone this kind of testing.)

And there's the British–South African swimmer Lewis Pugh, who is nicknamed the Sir Edmund Hillary of swimming. He has swum in the Arctic, in a meltwater lake on Mount Everest, and in Antarctica's Ross Sea. Scientists studying Pugh have found that his core body temperature rises even *before* he hits the water, reaching temperatures as high as one hundred and one degrees Fahrenheit. Professor Tim Noakes, a sports physiologist from the University of Cape Town, South Africa, first noted this response. In the *Lancet,* he called it "anticipatory thermogenesis": the creation of heat before an event. It's Pugh's Pavlovian response, from years of cold-water conditioning.

As for the rest of us, what happens to our bodies in cold water? I ask Hirofumi Tanaka, the longevity researcher, if there are any long-term studies of cold-water swimming and health. "We know the response, the diving reflex, when you put your face in cold water—the blood vessels in your skin constrict and your heart rate drops like crazy," he says. "But we don't have a lot of research in terms of chronic exposure to exercise in the cold." Then he tells me about the *ama*.

A couple of years ago, Tanaka went back to Japan to study the *ama*, the legendary female free divers of Japan and Korea. *Ama* is Japanese for "women of the sea." Carrying on this region's more than two-thousand-year-old tradition of hunting for shellfish, the women begin diving at age thirteen or fourteen; the group Tanaka studied was composed of sixty-five-year-olds on average. Like the Moken sea nomads of Southeast Asia, the *ama* pass on their skills and knowledge about the importance of the sea in stories told over generations. As with the Moken children, the practice of diving for shellfish changes their physical bodies, too. They dive up to two hundred times a day, every day, year-round. When it comes to vascular function, Tanaka says, they are "sky-high."

The *ama* are exposed to the diving reflex on a daily basis, hundreds of times a day. Tanaka had wondered if the *ama*'s arterial structure and function had adapted to resemble that seen in other diving mammals. He found that the women had significantly lower heart rates and less arterial stiffness when compared to other adults living in the same fishing village. They did, however, suffer from hearing loss—fifty years of exposure to cold water has adverse effects, too.

The scientific picture is far from complete, but there's a growing body of research on the therapeutic benefits of immersing ourselves in water. Warm-water immersion has its perks, too—studies show that one-hour head-out immersion in ninety-degree water lowers heart rate and blood pressure, promoting relaxation. But immersion in fifty-seven-degree water for the same period boosts the metabolic rate by 350 percent and dopamine by 250 percent. And when it comes to actually swimming in that water, other research shows that regular cold-water winter swimming significantly reduces tension, fatigue, and pain among participants—and improves general well-being.

I need to look no further than the Dolphin Club's own archives for convincing snapshots of swimming health. Back in 1974, Jack LaLanne—he of the famed fitness empire—swam while towing a rowboat behind him from Alcatraz to the club in less than ninety minutes, *all with his legs shackled and his arms manacled.* In a black-and-white photo from that day, the astonishingly robust LaLanne holds up his handcuffed (and well-muscled) wrists in triumph as he nears Aquatic Park. He was sixty years old. When LaLanne was seventy, shackled and manacled again, he swam a mile and a half in Long Beach Harbor, towing seventy boats with seventy passengers.

LaLanne swam every day. No surprise, then, that he was made an honorary lifetime member of the Dolphin Club. He died in 2011, at the age of ninety-six.

On a more contemporary morning at Aquatic Park, the cold water sloshing around our shoulders, I ask Kim if she thinks certain bodies tend to do better in the bay. New research into human physical performance shows that elite swimmers, unlike elite runners, can excel with different body types across all distances; an analysis of runners in the 2012 London Olympics revealed that 200-meter sprinters were significantly larger than marathoners, but the corresponding 50-meter-freestyle pool sprinters, for example, shared a similar body mass with 10,000-meter-open-water marathoners, regardless of height or sex. All bodies can do well in water, it seems. But what about when the water is cold? "Well, the theory is that you get more brown fat from being in cold water," Kim explains, as we pause to tread water and chat. "Brown fat burns energy and generates heat, and white fat doesn't." She laughs and shrugs. "Or so I'm told."

NOT LONG AFTER that swim, I drive five miles to the south, cross a bridgeway to a soaring futuristic building with rooftop gardens overlooking Golden Gate Park, and duck into the office of Dr. Shingo Kajimura to talk to him about what fat, cold water, and health could possibly have to do with each other. He's a prize-winning biochemist at the University of California, San Francisco, who runs a lab that is trying to engineer the way fat cells fight obesity and metabolic disease. A boyish man with a relaxed manner and a ready smile, Kajimura is fascinated by how animals adapt to their environment. As a kid growing up in the Tokyo suburbs, his job was to catch fish for dinner: sardines, say, or flounder. If he wasn't a scientist, he says, he'd be a fisherman and a sushi chef in San Francisco.

His early curiosity about fish adaptations—how salmon can swim from freshwater to saltwater, for example, or how catfish can thrive in dirty water—led to an interest in how mammals could adapt to cold conditions. "I was living in Michigan back then. I thought about cold all the time," he admits. But it was serendipitous, because it got him interested in the cutting-edge science of fat.

Kajimura tells me a tale of two fats: Humans, like other mammals, are born with two kinds of fat. White fat stores energy. Brown fat burns it, creating heat energy. Cold-water swimming is a combination of chronic cold exposure and exercise, both of which are known to have a "browning" effect on white fat—turning it into what's called beige fat—and revving up your metabolism.

Metabolism, of course, is a hot topic. Kajimura gets calls all the time from gyms in LA and New York. "They say, 'We'd like to start yoga in the cold—is that good for you?'" he says, laughing. "I say, 'It depends.' Exercising in the cold is good for some people, but not others." He knows that it's not a neat or satisfying answer, but—well, that's science.

White fat cells are almost 90 percent lipid—it's where our stores of energy live, says Kajimura. Brown fat cells, by contrast, are among the most mitochondria-rich cells in the human body—they are our fuel-burning engines. In the lab's studies with mice, exercise induced the browning of white fat, which was increased further by cool temperatures; this beige fat protected the mice from obesity and diabetes, and they were able to stay lean and healthy even when fed a high-fat diet. But because the science is so new—brown fat was only proven to exist in human adults in 2009—the molecular level of these processes is not yet clear.

Babies are born with lots of brown fat. "Since babies don't have enough muscle to shiver when they're cold to generate heat, brown fat is very important to regulate body temperature," Kajimura explains. He shows me a scientific illustration: a human infant, shaded with brown areas on the back and neck, where brown fat deposits are rich. The major coverage area resembles nothing so much as a winter scarf draped around the neck.

But there's a dramatic decline in brown fat when we reach our fifties and sixties, and it correlates neatly with age-related obesity. "Most people gain weight at this time, and it's not because they're eating more," Kajimura says. "It's very fascinating to us. You gain weight because your energy expenditure goes down. We don't fully understand why, but we speculate that the loss of brown fat contributes to it. What are the factors? Can we reverse the gain by creating new types of energy-burning brown fat even after you lose it?"

Cold exposure results in a stress response in our bodies: when you feel cold, your body compensates with blood flow, and blood vessel formation and circulation. But while the cold is one of the most efficient ways to burn energy— even more than exercise is—it's lousy for your heart, because cold stimulates vasoconstriction, and your blood pressure goes up. "Old people get strokes early in the morning in the wintertime," Kajimura tells me. "Cold exposure is beneficial to healthy people but not for people with heart trouble. It's the same for exercise—weight lifting or intense exercise is not good for you if you have cardiovascular risk. We can't apply or generalize this as a therapy for everyone. It depends on your age, how healthy you are, your family history."

But Kajimura finds the synergistic health pairing of swimming and cold water a tantalizing idea. "When I was a kid in Japan, my grandmother would send me outside to play in the wintertime," he recalls. Her command: Kids had to play outside in the cold. Take off a shirt, she said, and that would keep the doctor away.

"I've talked to people in Siberia, Russia—they jump into cold water all the time," Kajimura says, a bit wonderingly. "It's terrible from a cardiovascular standpoint, but people realize that there is something good about this—immunity, viral resistance. But we're not sure why that is." The specific mechanisms are still not completely understood, but evidence is accumulating.

In 2012, Russia held its first winter ice swimming competition in the middle of a frozen lake in Tyumen, a town in the vast region of Siberia. Organizers cut four 25-meter lap lanes into the ice. Swimmers flew in from all over the world to compete; the Israeli ice swimmer Ram Barkai, who lives in South Africa and founded the International Ice Swimming Association in 2009 to standardize cold open-water swimming, was one of them.

Faced with the astounding cold on the first day of competition, Barkai and his fellow swimmers suppressed "an extremely strong urge to drink ourselves silly," he writes in an account of that day. On the second day, the air was minus twenty-two degrees Fahrenheit—wet towels left out after the previous day's races froze and stood straight at attention. The water temperature held at the freezing point, thirty-two degrees. Just before Barkai was called back for his one-kilometer heat, he watched a Russian woman finish her endurance swim, swimming breaststroke with her head up, without goggles.

"Her eyelashes froze solid and she couldn't open them," writes Barkai. "They basically dragged her to the sauna to slowly defrost her eyes. Moisture in the nose froze solid. Breathing was like inhaling wasabi in slow shallow intakes. Any facial hair or long hair exposed to the icy air just froze immediately." Yet he notes that the water looked surprisingly inviting.

Barkai describes the post-race prize—skin lobster-red, body uncontrollably shivering—as the feeling of being intensely, vigorously alive: "The cold and the swim gives one such a rush and sense of health and vigor which is hard to explain unless you have done it."

When I get him on the phone from his home in South Africa to ask him about ice swimming for wellness, Barkai laughs. "Some people would argue that this is extreme *un*-wellness," he says. "I've been told by so many doctors I should have been dead long ago." But he continues to chase ice around the world, in pursuit of his "mad sport," for the heightening experience that he describes in his account of that day in Siberia. He recently returned from another swim in the same place and wants me to know that a decade of ice swimming has only made him feel more robust.

By the beginning of 2018, more than two hundred and fifty people had swum a certified "ice mile"—a mile or more in forty-one-degree water or colder.

Back in Kajimura's office, we marvel at the idea of swimming in a pool cut into the Siberian ice. "I guess whatever doesn't kill you makes you stronger," Kajimura says thoughtfully. "I used to think it was all philosophical, but it might be true from a clinical standpoint."

A glossary of common (and not-so-common) health ailments associated with swimming:

swimmer's ear: a bacterial or fungal infection of the outer ear canal brought on by water that stays in the ear after swimming (treated with ear drops to reduce inflammation and fight infection).

exostosis: an abnormal growth of bone within the ear canal that is caused by frequent exposure to cold water and windy conditions, often affecting surfers and divers (once the growth blocks the ear canal, the condition requires surgery).

cryptosporidiosis: a gastrointestinal and respiratory illness caused by a hardy, chlorine-resistant parasite, and the most common infection at pools and water parks (most people with healthy immune systems recover without treatment);

sea lice: stinging microscopic jellyfish larvae that often get trapped in the space between skin and swimsuit, causing itchy rashes and blisters (corticosteroids or antihistamines can help alleviate the severity of symptoms).

tinea pedis, or athlete's foot: common in damp locker rooms and swimming pools the world over, caused by a fungus that results in a scaly red rash (treated with antifungal medication).

Legionnaires' disease: a severe form of pneumonia caused by the *Legionella* bacterium when it contaminates swimming pools, hot tubs, whirlpools, and other water systems (prompt treatment with antibiotics is critical).

tendinitis, or swimmer's shoulder: a common inflammation of the fibrous cords connecting muscle to bone around the shoulder joint due to repetitive motions (cross-training, stretching, strength training, and rest are recommended).

swimming-induced pulmonary edema: a sudden onset of excess fluid in the lungs that results in difficulty breathing and may be related to strenuous swimming and cold-water immersion (treatment includes oxygen therapy and monitoring).

green hair (it's a thing!): results from the reaction of chlorine with copper and other hard metals found in pool water; green-tinged oxidized metals are absorbed by hair (baking soda can help).

cercarial dermatitis, or swimmer's itch: a rash caused by an allergic reaction to burrowing parasites common in ducks and other birds that dwell in freshwater lakes and ponds (calamine and antihistamines can reduce itching, but believe you me, they don't do much).

YOU CAN CALL me the Bumpy Bride. My husband does. You can't see it in the pictures, but a decade ago, at the very moment of our heartfelt declarations before a hundred of our closest friends and family, my skin was completely covered in a fine, full-body rash. Head to (miserably itching) toe.

On that bright summer afternoon, we were married on a spit of land overlooking Lake George, in the Adirondack Mountains near the New York–Vermont border. It's a lake known for its pristine water—so clean that New York State classifies it as drinking water. The bumps were an allergic reaction to the microscopic parasites that normally live in the waterfowl that frequent that lake—the rashy horror that is swimmer's itch.

I've endured all manner of welts to do what I love: swimming in Australia, surfing in Mexico, scuba diving in Panama. I've visited mosquito-filled Arctic summer beaches and sandfly-infested Hawaiian beaches. Always I return bearing itchy red badges of courage. Swimmer's itch. I try to own it: the swimming comes first, the suffering second. Still, these bugs define me somehow. In his wedding vows, my husband declared before witnesses that he could not promise to protect me from the "biting, stinging creatures of land and sea." But he promised to try.

Diana Nyad swam from Cuba to Florida and emerged unrecognizable because of jellyfish stings to her face. Lynne Cox was the first to swim in so many places, among them the Cape of Good Hope, patrolled by sharks and sea snakes. Martin Strel, the Slovenian "hero in a Speedo," swam the piranha-infested Amazon—all three thousand three hundred miles of it—risking the most agonizing of deaths by parasites, stingrays, and bull sharks.

Most of the aforementioned are warm-water afflictions, which I guess is a kind of luck, because at the very least I can retreat to other, colder waters, like those of San Francisco, which might just be specifically salutary to a swimmer like me.

WITH ALL THIS talk of how cold-water swimming can be good for you, I decide that I've got to lose the wetsuit. If eighty-year-old Mimi can do it, and with such aplomb, I should at least try it, right?

Another early morning at the Dolphin Club, this time in mid-March. In the midst of a colossal downpour, the water temperature in the bay has ticked up to an almost balmy fifty-six degrees. Somehow it seems to always be raining when I go open-water swimming, which makes for the unfortunate circumstance of clammy arrivals and departures. There isn't a soul in the water when I get to Aquatic Park to assess the conditions. I wonder if the reports of thunder and lightning are keeping swimmers away. But then Kim drives up and hops excitedly out of her car, a black Land Rover. "Whoo!" she crows. On her advice, I go to stash a thermos of hot ginger tea in my locker for drinking in the sauna post-swim. "It'll help warm you up afterward," she says. "But don't worry, you'll do great!"

A steady stream of swimsuit-clad bodies rolls with us out of the locker rooms and onto the sand. South Enders mingle convivially with Dolphin Clubbers as everyone discusses the conditions while standing knee-deep in the lapping water. (When I ask one swimmer, a middle-aged woman named Kate, how she'd characterize the two clubs, she confides that the Dolphin Club is "like living with your parents—we're more conservative. The South End is like the frat house. They're more risky." Standing next to Kate is her friend, a South Ender, who laughs appreciatively at this.)

Kim proudly proclaims my maiden voyage to anyone within earshot: "This is Bonnie. She's swimming without a wetsuit today for the first time!" I wave weakly. After a chorus of hellos, introductions, and a bit of trash talk, they all set off, one by one. Then it's my turn. I give the inside surface of my goggles one last swipe with my thumbs, steel my core muscles, and take the plunge.

Immediately, as I stroke through the first hundred yards, the surface of my skin starts generating a peculiar prickly heat—it's a kind of ice fire, flaming its way all over my body. It lasts for about sixty seconds. And then—well, I feel fine. We swim around Hyde Park Pier and turn parallel to the shore, following a line of buoys west across the cove toward Aquatic Park Pier. Our swim is punctuated every now and again by Kim's signature whoops—every dozen breaths or so, to mark her enthusiasm for the whole venture.

More than once, Kim has told me that there's a high to being in the rousingly crisp water, "with just what we came into the world with and a bit of Lycra." And it's true—in my skin, I feel more than fine. I feel great, amazing, *alive*. The sky clears. We pause at the far side buoy, the one planted with a flag and a thermometer, to check in with each other. Other swimmers join us at the flag, and as we tread water together, it's like a little tea party out there. By then, I don't feel the cold at all. "We'll take it easy since it's your first time," Kim cautions. "I know you can swim longer, but you'll get after-drop. Your body temperature will keep dropping after you get out, and that's when you'll get really cold." Turns out when it comes to cold, the biggest threat isn't the swim itself but the afterdrop that follows.

On the buoy trail back to the club, I alternate between freestyle and breaststroke, enjoying the view of the sandy beach and its swimmers. Still, at the edge of my conscious-ness, there's a little lurking worry. I can't help but think about Guðlaugur in the freezing North Atlantic, and of John Aldridge, the lobsterman from Long Island, my own home island: in 2013, Aldridge fell overboard in the middle of the night off the coast of Montauk and survived the next twelve hours in seventy-two-degree water by using his green rubber boots as flotation devices. What must it have been like to be out there for so long, in the cold? They were accidental swim-mers in their cold-water ordeals, and here we are doing it for fun. My twenty-five-minute maiden journey is over like that, with a tidal adrenaline rush. But as we hit the beach, my left pinky finger starts to separate from the rest of my hand in a clawlike configuration, almost as a warning.

In the shower, the afterdrop arrives. I furiously crank the faucet toward *H*, but I can't get warm or stop shivering no matter how far I turn the knob. My teeth chatter. As I rub my arms and legs, my jaw begins to clench.

The Dolphin Club, as it happens, is where longtime member Thomas Nuckton, an intensive care specialist, made a sideline of studying hypothermia and afterdrop in his fellow swimmers. The current U.S. Coast Guard immersion survival tables and computer programs actually reference one of Nuckton's studies, which quantifies a shipwreck survivor's biophysical parameters with methods that were developed with Dolphin Club swimmers. His work over the past two decades illustrated the afterdrop phenomenon: body temperatures continue to go down even after swimmers get out of the water, and mild hypothermia, a couple of degrees below normal, is fairly common. The takeaway: open-water swimmers, especially beginners, would be well advised to take it easy and carefully monitor their bodies' responses, especially after a swim is over. In a 2015 study of experienced ice-mile swimmers, Swiss researchers who followed in Nuckton's footsteps found that hypothermia didn't actually set in until after the participants had finished their swims.

Finally, after about ten minutes in the sauna, nestled in the warm conversation and camaraderie that thrives there, I begin to regain control of my extremities. And as I go about the rest of my day—to a café for breakfast with Kim, and then off to meet a writing buddy—I feel a secret pride in my accomplishment. Later, I walk along the waterfront and observe the moody bay with its damp and flickering light. *Today I swam out there with no wetsuit*, I think. I smile to myself, newly attuned and alert to the pulse of the bay as an echo of my own.

Why did I do it? I realize that it's because I want to knock on heaven's door and have a chat with the devil, too.

I have been afraid of death since I was very small. I remember visiting my great-grandfather's grave in Brooklyn during the spring Qingming festival, when Taoists honor their dead with ancestral grave sweeping. We burned incense and joss-paper ingots so my *bok-gung* could have ghost money to spend in heaven. What defined those visits for me, though, was not the story of what we were doing and why we were doing it. It was fear. Fear of the dark, inexplicable unknown; fear of *not being*. That deep anxiety over dying has stuck with me. Even though I am now grown, it's what jolts me awake in the night.

Swimming in open water is one small way of confronting that—of getting closer to the fire of wanting to stay alive, of warding off death, without the terror of having to do it for real. Maybe it's a kind of dress rehearsal. The sea is a deep, alien place. There's an energy to it, an element of danger that requires a giving over of the self, that makes swimming in heavy water a kind of sacrament. It is a suitable environment to engage with the deep strangeness of the human mind and its fears. Our feet are taken out from underneath us; there are unknowable fathoms below. There are moments of terror. Safety is restored when we set foot on land again back in San Francisco. Though I shiver upon emerging, with the accomplishment comes a powerful sense of hale and hardy vigor, of physical fortitude. And gratitude, quite simply, that I get to feel this at all.

Now, every time I drive on the Bay Bridge, along the waterfront, or over the Golden Gate Bridge, I pause to reconsider the bay. For a few minutes each morning on the way to my office in San Francisco, I might lose myself in the landscape. Or I might see the evening water shelled with pink and wonder how it felt earlier that day. Was it charged with cold, or had the sun warmed it enough to give one's entry something like a velvety comfort?

7

Open Water, Meet Awe

We submerge ourselves in the natural world because the natural world has a way of eliciting awe. Every morning at seven a.m. in Sydney, Australia, hundreds of swimmers gather at the city's famous Manly Beach for an open-water swim. They swim about half a mile across a bay to Shelly Beach. Then they turn around and swim back. The locals describe it as their "wake-up call."

The swimmers wear bright pink swim caps. The squad was started by middle-aged women who wanted to gain courage from each other to swim that distance across the open water. In an essay about her daily outings with the group, the Australian writer and broadcaster Julia Baird observes the way they watch the scroll of scenery as they swim: "Most days, at some spot along the mile-long route, heads will cluster, arms pointing down under the water at enormous blue groupers, white dolphins, color-changing cuttlefish, wobbegongs . . . even tiny turtles and sea horses." Of the gangs of dusky whale sharks that swim beneath, Baird takes note: "There's a reason a collective term for sharks is a shiver."

Some days the swimmers are lashed by jellyfish and currents and powerful surf. (When I was a college student studying abroad in Sydney, I swam frequently at Manly and can attest to the unpleasantness of the jellyfish.) Some days the whales come. It's akin to a religious experience.

"As your arms circle, swing, and pull along the edge of a vast ocean, your mind wanders," Baird writes. With the drift into deeper waters comes freedom and the shift in perception that is awe. "Awe," she continues, "experienced when you witness something astonishing, unfathomable, or greater than yourself, ventilates and expands our concept of time."

We feel light, suspended. Time slows down in the best way, and we feel that we have more of it. Psychologists at Stanford University and the University of Minnesota, led by researcher Melanie Rudd, have shown that after experiencing awe, we are more likely to help others and to be relaxed and satisfied with life. When I ask Rudd about her findings, she explains that the experience of awe heightens our focus on the present. "It captivates people's attention with what is currently happening with them and around them," she says. And the effects of awe are striking even beyond the moment—it makes us feel more time-rich, less impatient, more generous. It helps us to be our better selves. And who doesn't want that?

Back on the other side of the Pacific in San Francisco, Kim and I are swimming one morning when a seagull pegs me on the shoulder, mid freestyle stroke. I nearly jump out of my swimsuit in surprise, and then I call out to Kim. "I think a bird just *hit* me," I exclaim, incredulous.

"It's *their* swimming pool," Kim answers, laughing. "We're just the fools who think we can swim in it."

SWIMMING IS, BY our human definition, a constant state of not drowning. *The Oxford English Dictionary* emphasizes the propulsion of the body through water with one's limbs and a position afloat on the water's surface. To drown is to die through immersion or submersion—the body *under* the surface—in water and inhalation of that water. We know from the most ancient of times that the boundary between the two states of being is thin; it grows permeable when we're not looking.

A friend turns me on to Loudon Wainwright III's 1973 classic "The Swimming Song." It's all about the quintessential experience of summer swimming in oceans, pools, and public reservoirs. Wainwright celebrates the whoop-of-joy freedom that swimming grants us. And yet even this buoyant song reminds us of the boundary line:

> This summer I went swimming
> This summer I might have drowned
> But I held my breath and I kicked my feet
> And I moved my arms around

Then it continues:

> I salt my wounds, chlorine my eyes
> I'm a self-destructive fool

There's caution here. And yet we dance near that line anyway, because there's something there to see.

In the documentary *Fishpeople*, filmmaker Keith Malloy interviews surfers, spearfishers, swimmers, and others to create a vivid picture of how their lives are transformed by the sea. These are people who live in the water for all of its sensory immediacy and also for the outlook it fosters. At some point or another, they all feel compelled to speak about how the ocean brings them to a hyperawareness of our precarious existence.

The young Tahitian Matahi Drollet, who grew up surfing the storied Teahupo'o surf break, is shown blasting through some of the biggest barrels he'd ever surfed there—including the ride that garnered him worldwide acclaim when it was caught on film and won an award sponsored by Billabong in 2015. He was sixteen years old. His commentary on the vivid experience of this wave? "I thought I was gonna die," he says, with a little disbelieving laugh.

In another scene from the film, the champion spearfisher Kimi Werner, who grew up in Oahu and learned free diving and spearfishing from her father, swims calmly with a huge shark, holding on to its dorsal fin for a spell before departing back to the surface. "It is dangerous. I *am* scared," she says of all the time she spends underwater. She remembers her dad telling her this if she ever got scared: *Just relax—and remember how to swim.*

Another of Malloy's subjects is Lynne Cox, a hero to so many swimmers, including Kim. Cox, of course, holds dozens of major open-water records; in 1977, she was the first to swim around the Cape of Good Hope in South Africa, entering the water by climbing down a sheer cliff and into surging twenty-foot surf that repeatedly threw her back to the sand. I ask her about how open water has shaped her world view. She says that she equates being in the ocean with "an acute awareness of your life, in the moment." You go out there expecting something new, but you don't necessarily know what that will be. Being in the pool, going back and forth, is not the same. "Being in the ocean," Cox tells me, "you could become part of the food chain at any moment."

The understanding of this adjacency, this porousness between states of being, can be comforting. When the pioneer Australian surfer Dave Rastovich describes being in the ocean as "meaningful play"—whether it's swimming, surfing, or floating on an inflatable raft—I get it. "When my dad died, I just kept going in the ocean," he says—it was what made the difference in his acceptance of life and death.

KIM REMEMBERS SWIMMING seventeen miles across Cook Strait, a stretch of water between the North and South Islands of New Zealand, with a pod of dolphins. It was her first real solo expedition, in March 2012, and the first of her successful Oceans Seven endurance swims. Her grandfather was in ill health, and she felt that it would mean something to return to her home turf and swim in his honor.

As a girl, Kim spent summer holidays at the beach with her grandparents, who were farmers. She was close with her grandfather, whom she called Poppa. What the ocean recalls for her more than anything is sitting contentedly in the waves, being sunburned as hell, and not even knowing until the next day the degree of the burn. Her grandparents would shout when it was time to go to the ice cream store. The days felt endless. When she swims now, she feels a sensory connection to a time in her youth when there was that freedom.

In the Cook Strait, Kim's boat pilot told her that one in six swimmers encounters sharks. She was anxious, but mid-swim, dolphins showed up. It was the first time she'd ever had the experience of swimming with them. "They were squeaking around me, like, *The cavalry is here!*" she remembers. She chirped back excitedly, channeling her inner twelve-year-old. The dolphins zipped around and below, escorting her for just under an hour. She didn't see any sharks out in the strait, and she thinks it was because the dolphins were protecting her.

Afterward, Kim beelined to her grandfather's bedside. "What I'm most proud of is being able to lie next to Poppa and show him the video of me swimming the Cook Strait with the dolphins," Kim tells me. He'd fought in World War II and suffered from post-traumatic stress, but animals and nature both calmed him. Kim was grateful to be able to share her swim with him. He could no longer talk, but he smiled at her to let her know he'd heard. Not long afterward, he died in his home.

A few months after his death, Kim swam the Molokai Channel, between the Hawaiian islands of Molokai and

Maui. At the end of that swim, she saw and heard humpback whales singing at her. "In Hawaii, they call that *aumakua*— that's your ancestors speaking to you," she tells me. There were dolphins on that swim, too. The energy they brought made her feel like they were all in it together, that she wasn't alone. It felt primal. She could taste the life in the water; she could smell the diesel from the boat next to her. She concentrated on her hands in front of her. At night, the bioluminescence emitted by tiny marine creatures fluttered off her fingertips like glitter. Focusing on her fingers was meditative. It made her feel safe. The clarity of the water soothed her; the deep breathing steadied her.

In the essay "I Will Always Inhabit the Water," the writer Lidia Yuknavitch describes swimming as being defined in large part by "the great intake of air, a breath that keeps a human able to move through water as if we were not gone from our breathable blue past." You can read this as a yearning for that breathable blue past—and what swimmer among us has not longed for this—but you can also read it as an affirmation of what keeps us *us*: the air we breathe, the air we *need*, even as we put our faces in the water.

SOMETHING ABOUT THE rhythm of how we breathe while we're in the water changes us. Deep breathing research is in its infancy, but we know that this pace of breath is soothing—there's a feedback loop between our breathing patterns and the nerve centers that fire our anxiety responses. When we're stressed, we tend to take short, rapid breaths; if we breathe deeply and slowly, that counteracts the stress and dampens our alarm system. In this way, our arousal and breathing centers are reciprocally linked. Swimming is particular in its activation of deep breathing. It's the nature of the exercise: you take a big breath, hold it, and then release it slowly.

Kim has unusually large lungs, perhaps the ideal bellows for big, slow breaths. On the day we first met, she showed me the spot above her collarbone where an acupuncturist once poked a needle into her lung by accident and collapsed it. Those lungs carry her far when it comes to expedition swims.

The breaths, then, make swimming like moving meditation. We take a breath. We hold. We pull, and glide. We take another breath. In between breaths, the thinking happens— about each stroke, each kick, each breath. As we become better swimmers, there is less conscious thinking about swimming and our thoughts are released, free to wander as they may. All the while, the body works. We notice things: how the water moves, what the temperature is like, whether the swimming feels easy or difficult. We are at once hyper-aware and loosed from our bodily constraints.

"Swimming in water is the only state of being I know where I feel free," writes Yuknavitch. A former competitive swimmer, she has written at length about swimming for well-being, especially as she ages. Water, she says, helps a body remember that life and time are fluid: "I look a little lumbering and soft, aged and lumpy. But put me in water . . .

put me in water for even ten seconds, and I will prove to you that a body is anything you want it to be."

I ask Tanaka, the longevity researcher, what makes swimming so good for aging bodies. Weightlessness, he says. Physical activity without the pain and damage of land-based impact. Coolness, and buoyancy, to reduce inflammation and support the body. And one more thing, the most important thing.

"I will tell you the one thing that distinguishes swimming from all other forms of exercise." I listen carefully. "People enjoy it a lot more." I wait. *That's it?* He goes on to relate something we all know in our bones to be true: Tons of us have New Year's resolutions to exercise; after six months, half of us drop out. But this is where swimming has a huge benefit and advantage. "We do assessments of mood state," Tanaka explains. "And with identical exercise programs in running, cycling, and swimming, people place the highest enjoyment in swimming." In other words, people keep swimming because they *like* it. Swimming is the second most popular recreational activity in America, outranked only by walking. But swimming is the one that quite literally takes us out of our element.

We swim, and we get out from under the thumb of the everyday. "There's a giddiness to being in that water," Kim observes. "It connects with a playfulness that we forget about as adults." I think about the way that the serious-looking older man in the pool this morning dove under the lanes on his way out, spiraling down to the bottom, arms out-stretched, as if he had all the time in the world. And I think about children in the pool during afternoon family swim, their elation so palpable. Swimming is a way for us to remember how to play.

Once, in thick autumn darkness while sailing around the islands off the coast of British Columbia, I jumped off the back of the boat and into the unknown—the icy water in that moment looked impenetrably black—just for the chance to make a phosphorescent snow angel. Clouds of glowing bio-luminescence bloomed around me as I treaded water, a kind of aquatic light show. When I climbed out of the water and rubbed my arms vigorously, sparks flew.

This is the wonder for which we immerse ourselves, says the surfer Dave Rastovich: "We forget our bodies as we know them and we just . . . swim."

YEARS AGO, A close friend and I cemented a friendship that began in college by splashing our way around Hawaii, start-ing on his home island of Oahu. We visited other islands, too, like Kauai, where we waded into the Pacific at Polihale Beach, a remote seventeen-mile stretch of white sand at the end of the long, rutted dirt road that seemed as far away as you can get from anywhere.

We swam in that heaving body of aquamarine, and what I remember most is the profound feeling that the ocean water had weight. In the years since, I've come to appreciate open water—an ocean, a lake big enough to generate its own waves—as its own animal. I see swimming as a way to get to know a place with an intimacy that I otherwise wouldn't have.

The pleasures of swimming in a place can be everyday, routine, familiar. In 1779, a lieutenant of Captain James Cook's admired the native Hawaiians' swimming abilities with an entry in his ship's log: "The Women could swim off to the Ship, & continue half a day in the Water"; in Hawaiian, Polynesian, and other enduring island cultures of the Pacific, he observed, the men, women, and children seemed "almost amphibious" from birth. This is as lovely a description of the freewheeling freedom of swimmers as any I have come across.

I feel that freedom when I'm swimming in San Francisco Bay, but I am just as aware of the hazards that are ever present at its edges. Because of the cold, there's another layer of intensity to the open-water experience. "You don't belong here," Kim tells me, matter-of-factly, "but you do it anyway." With the cold, the swim is like a fire drill for your body. "It's fight or flight that's engaged when you're in that water," she explains. "Everything is telling you that you shouldn't be doing what you're doing. And yet you still do it." Some of the benefits of swimming derive, ironically, from daring to come as close as we can to this very fight for survival. That's the sublime: the awe and the terror, together. Those moments of panic, the electric flashes of fear, are elucidating, exhilarating. The act of getting in is a small defiance of death itself.

In her 1937 essay "Undersea," Rachel Carson eloquently described the ocean as a tangible way for humans to contemplate the vast interconnectedness of life. "Individual elements are lost to view, only to repair again and again in different incarnations in a kind of material immortality," she wrote. It doesn't matter if it's the ear bones of whales or the teeth of sharks. "Against this cosmic background the lifespan of a particular plant or animal appears, not as drama complete in itself, but only as a brief interlude in a panorama of endless change." We're all connected in this vastness, and our presence in the sea is but a blip, a shout into the void.

We shout anyway.

To what lengths will one person go to chase the sublime? Back in the sauna at the Dolphin Club, Kim is cooking up plans to be the first person ever to swim the Oceans Seven *and* climb the Seven Summits. It's a thrilling prospect, not least because she will have to rely on that right leg again to carry her up those peaks. She has made practice runs up two fourteeners—fourteen-thousand-foot-plus mountains, that is—in California and Colorado. She still spends her mornings swimming. The only difference is that she now spends her evenings climbing the StairMaster.

In October 2017, she sends me a text, and I reflexively whoop out loud when I read it: she has just climbed to the top of Mount Kilimanjaro, the first of her summits. As she powers through the next few months—knocking off Australia's Mount Kosciuszko in December and Mount Aconcagua, in the Andes, in January—she dives headfirst into mountaineering training. She hits the gym several times a week, carrying a fifty-pound backpack full of birdseed. She has Denali in her sights, and then Everest—she wants an all-female Sherpa team. Her next goal: to become known as the ultimate adventurer, of land as well as sea.

Swimming is the means that got her here, to even dream of such a thing. It healed her, body and soul, and brought her to a new state of exuberant health. At that moment in the sauna, Kim's goal was a secret—well, from the public, anyway. But she couldn't remember who else she'd told, so she asked everyone in the sauna to keep it close.

Though Kim first set off on her swim expeditions to regain a sense of self she'd lost—to revive herself, in the wake of almost losing a limb—over time that motivation changed. Through swimming, her focus gradually pulled back to take in the world beyond herself. She says there's nothing solo about a solo swim.

"There's a joy in making these swims bigger than myself," she says. Two of her last major swims had to do with bringing people together. In November 2016, she led a team of swimmers across the Dead Sea between Israel and Jordan— the first people ever to complete that swim—to highlight what the countries were doing to combat climate change in the region. "We were like a swimming science experiment," she says. "I had to put Vaseline in places I would never have dreamed of putting it. The salt burned my eyes like acid." But she would do it all again: Her goal was to get the Israeli and Jordanian governments to cooperate and let her do the swim. She succeeded.

The experience gave her heart and hope, six months later, to do the next swim. On Cinco de Mayo, 2017, Kim swam six miles around the existing border wall from the United States to Mexico, with a team of eleven other swimmers from around the world, from San Diego's Imperial Beach to Tijuana. They worked with the human rights organization Colibrí, which identifies people who have died in the crossing, no matter what the route. Her co-leader was the Mexican swimmer Antonio Argüelles; a few months later, he would go on to be just the seventh person, after Kim, to complete the arduous Oceans Seven open-water challenge.

Kim had the cooperation of the US Coast Guard and Customs and Border Patrol as well as the Mexican Navy—a colossal feat in this era of contentious border politics between the United States and Mexico. She phoned up everybody herself, emphatic that the swim was not about politics but about our common humanity.

As she swam up onto the beach in Tijuana, she saw more than a hundred Mexican schoolchildren on the cliff cheering and wearing T-shirts supporting the swim. Mother Teresa came to mind: "I alone cannot change the world, but I can cast a stone across the waters to create many ripples." It wasn't a bad metaphor, Kim thought, to understand the way that water connects us all: the commonality of it, the communality of it. She wants to make ripples.

Kim and the other swimmers were received in the water by the Mexican Navy, to process their paperwork. Their faces were radiant; they were feeling every emotion. Kim swam up to the boat, exhausted, but she grinned and asked, in a neighborly way, to great laughter, if she might borrow a cup of sugar.

COMMUNITY

◡

Beyond the wave they had gone through, they finally showed, side by side, still six feet apart, swimming shoreward with a steady stroke until the next wave should make them body-surf it or face and pierce it.

—JACK LONDON, "The Kanaka Surf"

The man floated in the pool, a speck of cool in a sea of hot. The brutal midday sun had burned off, leaving a lingering warmth in the desert air. Late afternoon, early evening—these were the best times to swim. If he looked up, he could see the palm-fringed canopy of the trees that lined the baroque, open-air pool, offering merciful shade to those seated at the edge. Turning his head, he could see the diving platforms of varying stratospheric heights and the exquisite handcrafted tile that lined the terrace. If he dove down, into the rich, layered blue depths, he could pretend he was in the Caribbean.

If, while floating, he held his head in a certain way, submerging his ears, he could avoid hearing the constant sound of firing practice: a percussive *pakapakapakapaka* that never let up.

Even though I know all about Green Sahara paleolakes by now, swimming in the desert still sounds like a kind of fever dream. The man, Joseph "Jay" Taylor, often felt that way himself. In Baghdad, which has been called the hottest place on earth, temperatures can exceed a hundred and twenty degrees in the summer months. But despite being surrounded by desert, Baghdad itself is a green city, situated along the winding Tigris River, its banks lined with willows, palms, and poplars.

At one of the serpentine bends in the river you will find Saddam Hussein's royal palace and its outdoor pool. The expansive swimming pool was commissioned by the dictator to please his two murderous sons, who were fond of swimming. It had an irregular bean shape, thirty-three yards at its longest, and a magnificent poolside decor that included dramatic lighted fountains, tall, leafy trees, and a pillared stone rotunda of heroic dimensions.

Between 2008 and 2010, Jay was stationed in Baghdad as a cultural attaché for the US Foreign Service. It was a volatile period in Iraq. The US Embassy was situated on the grounds of the royal palace—its official name was the Republican Palace, one of the many palaces and opulent homes that Hussein had built in strategic locations around the country (eighty-one, by one count). Each of them had a pool, an unequivocal sign of wealth in the desert. The Republican Palace was the residence where the dictator liked to entertain visiting heads of state. He himself did not live there, but it had two hundred and fifty-eight rooms and sprawling grounds. At the time Jay was there, the palace anchored the Green Zone, where the international community resided—military, diplomats, and civilians alike. It was deemed the safest place in Baghdad, though the first few months of Jay's tenure saw incessant shelling of the zone, with numerous casualties.

Here, the idea of an outdoor swimming pool seemed, to put it mildly, a little cuckoo. Especially one like this, adorned with eighteen-foot fountains and lighted with standing chandeliers for nighttime swimming. Jay couldn't believe that he got to swim in it, even if on more than one occasion he had to jump out of the deep end at the scream of an air-raid siren and, still dripping, clamber hastily into a concrete bunker as the *boom boom* of exploding mortars vibrated around him.

He swam every day, and he wasn't alone in his love for the pool. Daring soldiers made use of the tall diving platforms and posted their exploits on social media. But mostly people just liked to get in, paddle around a bit, sit at the edge, shoot the shit. Jay would occasionally see other swimmers doing laps. There was this one woman who served Joint Forces detail—she had a graceful freestyle stroke and, when she stopped to chat, a charmingly thick Australian accent.

The swimming lessons began one evening when Jay, after his workout, spotted his colleague Andry Rambolamanana. A tank of a man from Madagascar, Rambolamanana was an experienced kickboxer on land, but in the water he was flailing, thrashing so violently that Jay feared he might drown.

"Andry, what are you doing?" Jay asked him.

"Just swimming, boss!" Rambolamanana replied.

Jay offered to take on Rambolamanana as a student. Next he signed up Valya Krasteva, from Bulgaria, and Sandy

Yannick, also from Madagascar. Before long, strangers started inquiring at Jay's office about swim lessons, and he set up two beginner classes a week. Cooks, drivers, translators, peacekeeping troops, helicopter pilots: People from all over the world, from all kinds of places and backgrounds, wanted Jay to be their swim coach. Merlin Espinal, from Honduras; Indrani Pal, from India; Maka Beradze, from Ukraine; Mai Shahin, from Lebanon; J. P. Santana, from Mexico. It was a miniature United Nations, a global diaspora of people who had never learned to swim. They called him Coach Jay. And they called themselves the Baghdad Swim Team.

Coach Jay is a pen pal of mine. We began corresponding after he read an essay that I'd written about swimming as the last refuge from connectivity—the digital kind. He wrote to me to argue the opposite, that swimming is a way to form community, forge bonds, and find solace in a common pursuit. In 2009, he received an award from then Secretary of State Hillary Clinton for his service to the community in teaching all those wartime swimming lessons.

I wondered about all those people who ended up in Baghdad never having learned how to swim. And I wondered, how is it that some of us get to swim, and what stops those of us who don't? What forces keep us out of the water, and are they the same no matter where you come from?

This is about how swimming has brought us together, and how it has kept us apart.

8

Who Gets to Swim?

I n America, the pool is a privilege. People have historically had complicated feelings about water. Mixing in it
deliberately—as men and women, as rich and poor, as
black and brown and white—can stir up all kinds of fears.
As a society, we've kept different groups apart based on those
fears.

Public pools first proliferated in big cities like New York
and Chicago at the turn of the twentieth century. Throughout
the Progressive Era, swimming pools were places where
blacks, whites, and immigrants swam together, regardless
of race, in the interest of hygiene, writes the historian Jeff
Wiltse in *Contested Waters*, his engrossing social history of
the swimming pool in America. These early municipal pools
were in essence giant bathtubs for working-class neighborhoods; they also corralled rowdy, half-naked youths away
from public waterways, where they were perceived as nui-
sances (on a hot summer day, kids will be kids). Men and
women, though, were separated and swam on alternating
days.

By the 1920s things had changed: Cities began building larger recreational pools that were intended primarily for public leisure instead of public bathing. Men, women, and families were finally permitted to swim together, in the urban-led effort to encourage community socializing. Marquee pools included Fleishhacker Pool in San Francisco, a thousand-foot-long saltwater pool so gigantic that it required lifeguards in rowboats when it opened in 1925, and Astoria Pool, a grand art deco swimming and diving complex overlooking the East River between Queens and Manhattan that opened in 1936. Between the 1920s and the 1950s, tens of millions visited the country's municipal pools each year—and they did it for fun.

Coach Jay himself learned to swim as a boy at a YMCA in downtown Baltimore in the early 1950s, in an old tiled indoor pool that reverberated with the particular mayhem of children shouting and splashing in a confined space. It was the golden age of the Y, when young kids didn't have to wear swimsuits. At four years old, Jay was more comfortable swimming than walking. Swimming was important to his mother; the family took vacations to the glorious ten-mile stretch of beach in the resort town of Ocean City, Maryland.

Community swim clubs proliferated in the Baltimore suburbs, where Jay swam on his local team until he became a lifeguard. While in college at Tufts, studying government, he spent summers managing a pool in Baltimore. He taught lessons in swimming and lifesaving.

But during those same decades, the unprecedented mixing

of men and women in recreational pools intensified the old fears of interracial mixing. Though class lines had been erased at the pool, race lines hardened even further, resulting in riots and racial segregation. Black swimmers were attacked by white crowds in pools from Pittsburgh to St. Louis. At one Harlem pool in New York City, blacks and Puerto Ricans who lived just blocks away were deterred from entrance by the threat of violence by white swimmers.

In the 1950s and 1960s pools became sites of civil disobedience, and so did other aquatic spaces. Blacks across America protested being barred from public beaches with "wade-ins," showing up to swim en masse at all-white beaches by the ocean or the lake. At least one of these wade-ins, in Biloxi, Mississippi, ended in violence at the hands of a white mob; the Bloody Wade-In took place on Easter Sunday in 1960, on Biloxi's public beach. The question of beach access for blacks wasn't settled until eight years later, when a federal judge ruled that Mississippi's Gulf Coast beaches were open to everyone.

This was a fight not just for the right of access but for the right of recreation, of leisure, no matter what your skin color. Many activists saw pools and beaches as the ultimate symbols of that freedom. In the mingling of bodies, in the act of sharing the same water with others, you can read volumes. The volumes speak of acceptance. But when desegregation did happen, it wasn't always with the hoped-for results. In cities all across America, pools began to empty, and you can read that as a tragedy. "Between 1950 and 1970, millions of Americans chose to stop swimming at municipal pools," writes Wiltse. It was a "mass abandonment" of public space by white swimmers, accompanied by the construction of private club and backyard pools for those who could afford it. Social divisions, not surprisingly, became even more entrenched.

The historic lack of access to public pools also left America with a racial gap in swimming ability that persists today. Black children drown at a rate five times that of white children. And as with so many other things, money also has a heavy hand in the way swimmers are made: in the United States, nearly 80 percent of children in families with a household income of less than fifty thousand dollars have no or low swimming ability.

By the 1980s, when I was growing up on Long Island, suburban backyard pools had become the rule for families with means. As Wiltse puts it, backyard pools were installed because their owners "wanted to turn inward and privilege family over community," while more and more of America's numerous public pools, which provided for everyone else, were closed due to lack of use and funds. Many of them fell into disrepair.

My family was lucky enough to live not too far from one of these community pools, one that was not in disrepair. When I was eight years old, my parents gave me a choice: soccer or swim team. I chose swim team, as did my brother. Andy and I were tired of getting our shins kicked, and we didn't much like soccer, anyway. We spent the next ten years swimming with a scrappy local team two miles away. We loved not just swimming but also the kids we swam with. The feeling of belonging. This was our tribe. We made lasting friendships that crossed towns, cultures, and income brackets.

Unlike our own town, the Freeport pool was racially diverse. In that pool, there were brown and black bodies. In that pool, kids did not jam up the corners of their eyes with their fingers or make fun of my last name. In that pool, with all those other kinds of bodies, my body started to feel like mine in a way that was good.

Another thing about that team—it was coed. The original prohibitions at public pools were put in place in fear of this very thing: people of different races, genders, and backgrounds mixing together. For us, it was not so complicated as all that. Just puberty on the pool deck. Every day, we sipped from the heady cocktail of hormones and H_2O. Bodies simultaneously attracted and repelled, pulled and pushed, all invited to jump together into one chlorinated rectangle of possibility. This was freedom. It was a window open to the future, away from the strictures of home, parents, rules. Chlorine carried with it an appealing whiff of excitement. We could play at something we did not quite understand.

~

9

A Mini United Nations

J ay had been in Iraq just three days when he woke up in a daze and found his friend J. P. Santana's prosthetic arm on his doorstep. A second before, Jay had been juggling his first load of Baghdad laundry, depositing it in his FEMA trailer, just inside the complex that housed most of the embassy staff. Then came the mortar blast. It threw Jay against a wall, and he blacked out. It blew J.P.—who'd come by to collect Jay for dinner—thirty feet down the road, minus his arm.

J.P. yelled to Jay. "Let me hear your voice! I'm OK, are you OK?" Jay shouted back in the affirmative. J.P.'s own trailer was obliterated. A man across the street was killed.

If J.P. had been just a little bit later to Jay's door, "if he'd decided to shower," Jay says, "he would have been dead."

Amid the dust and debris, J.P. retrieved his prosthetic arm, and US Army Special Forces quickly arrived to seal off the trailer of the man who was killed. They carried the body away. J.P.'s trailer, still smoldering, was cordoned off. The troops told J.P. and Jay to come back in an hour. With nothing else to do but wait, the two men headed to dinner at the cavernous mess hall. Outside the door was an oil drum full of sand, into which armed personnel were required to discharge their weapons—*click click*—to show that they weren't loaded.

"The odd thing is, even the first time being in a bombing situation like that, we just get up and say, 'Oh, I hope they still have meatloaf,'" Jay tells me, shaking his head. "Because what can you do? You just pick up life and go on."

During times of war, people seek normalcy. Going to market, hosting dinner with friends, looking at baby pictures. I remember my friend's mother, who served as a combat nurse in Vietnam, saying that routine in the midst of chaos was important to her. Relationships were essential. "It was a way of showing the world," she told me, "that something vital hadn't yet been knocked out of us."

In 2008, five years after the US-led invasion of Iraq, Baghdad was unstable, despite a significant surge in troops to control sectarian violence. But still there was optimism: after decades of suspension, the Iraqi Fulbright program was resurrected, and Jay was tasked with finding promising young Iraqi intellectuals who were interested in completing advanced degrees in the United States. He flew to universities by helicopter, wearing a military helmet and a thirty-pound armored vest, because transport by air was far safer than traveling on the ground. Soldiers had to be in uniform at all times, outfitted in camouflage fatigues and carrying weapons, unless they were working out in the gym—or in the pool.

Jay spent many of his days in the palace's cavernous Green Room. A former reception hall, it was then serving as the office of public affairs. Among its most prominent features were fifty-foot ceilings and vainglorious portraits of Hussein, covered in tarps—and that glorious pool, glinting just outside. Jay's training as a public affairs officer included what to do in the building in case of attack. Use duct tape to stem bleeding. Cut out the carpet if needed to wrap any injured personnel; drag them out.

"The buildings were magnificent, monumental," Jay says. In person, he cuts a tidy figure. His sandy hair and mustache are carefully trimmed, and when I visit him in Maryland, his memories of Iraq are as precisely rendered as his facial hair. "Everything in the palace, even though lots of artifacts had been torn out before we got there, all the details were of the highest quality. The mill work, the lavatories, even the door hinges. The spaces were enormous, on the scale of the Library of Congress. Marble everything, chandeliers everywhere."

Jay split his time between the public affairs office and the cultural affairs section, located in another, smaller palace about two miles away. People called that one the "little palace." It, too, had a pool, supposedly put in by Hussein's sons. To cover ground between the two palaces, Jay rode a green Montague paratrooper folding bike—the same model that airborne soldiers used in Afghanistan; they could drop from a helicopter with it and ride off as soon as they landed. He didn't bother to wear a helmet.

Swimming has always been a means of escape: physical,

spiritual, mental. And if that's true, then what better place is there for a swim team than a war zone? Everyone had friends blown up and their own close calls. Near-death experiences are the kind of thing that knits you together. Get in a pool together afterward and, in the delayed-reaction realization that you're still alive, exuberance bubbles to the surface.

"The desert dust would create these gorgeous sunsets— the human instinct when you see one is to stop and look," Jay recalls of that time. "But what made it eerie in Baghdad is that it's also a wonderful time to mortar, because it means that when the US attack helicopters go looking for you, it's a little bit dusty, so they can't see you as well. So when it was an especially beautiful sunset, you could expect that mortars would fall."

That's the screwed-up logic of a combat zone.

COACH JAY BEGAN leading drills in the palace pool with Andry from Madagascar and Valya from Bulgaria, help- ing Andry to slow his frenetic windmill down and Valya to escape the tyranny of her archaic strokes.

Ten months into Jay's stay, the entire US community in the Green Zone moved from Hussein's palace into the just-completed and impressively fortified New Embassy Compound. The decision had been made to give the palace and the Green Zone back to the Iraqis; the hope was that both the palace and its pool would eventually be used by ordi- nary citizens. Though the move meant leaving the lavish pool behind, Jay found that the new facility had a twenty-five-yard indoor lap pool, open twenty-four hours a day. It was then that the swimming lessons began in earnest.

In the space of two weeks, Coach Jay's swimming students tripled, then doubled again: from four pupils to twelve, then twenty-four. Then they tripled and doubled some more. Andry and Valya brought their friends, and their friends brought *their* friends. Most were beginners, their skills raggedy but existent.

The back wall of the new pool was mostly glass, and outside, a Baghdad-modern version of the broad pedestrian esplanade connected housing blocks and offices to the gym and dining hall. From the walkway, you could see people swimming. "I guess we couldn't have asked for better advertising," says Jay. Andry worked in the cultural affairs section, too, assisting Jay with the Fulbright and other academic and professional exchange programs. The two men put up a few announcements around the Green Zone about the lessons, which were held three days a week, with morning and afternoon sessions.

A couple of months into the swimming experiment, Jay and Andry found themselves sitting in the office more than a little stunned at the overwhelming response to the lessons and wondering just what it was they'd started. The swim team was an all-volunteer effort on their part, organized in addition to their normal job duties. But as more swimmers joined, they felt compelled to hold enough classes to keep up with the numbers.

A new group of students appeared, people who had never before been in the water. A few of the Muslim women had never worn swimsuits in public. They told Jay that they'd never had the chance to do any sport except bowling. They arrived clutching Land's End catalogs and asked him what swimsuits to buy. Absent firsthand experience in the matter, Jay quickly referred all fashion questions to Indrani, his Bengali friend and colleague in the cultural affairs section, who helped each first-timer with the selection of a conservative two-piece or Speedo tank suit.

Jay gave every swimmer a number. In the earliest days, Valya was swimmer number one; Andry was number two. Every new swimmer was assigned a buddy already in the swim class. Everybody, even if experienced, would start off the same way: splashing water on their faces, blowing bubbles, pushing off the wall in a streamlined Superman pose. It built a culture of egalitarianism—it meant that someone who three weeks earlier was a beginner could then be in the position of teacher. Jay would be on deck or in the water, offering instruction; Andry, who quickly rose to deputy coach status, would do the same.

They played games to keep it entertaining. Jay taught life-saving and got inventive with his lesson plans. He loved old movies, and even old movies could form the basis for drills. "We'd play Guns of Navarone—you know, after that 1961 war movie with Gregory Peck?" he tells me. He'd have all the swimmers swim soundlessly, mostly submerged, with just their eyes above the water. Then he'd kill the lights at the pool, and he and Andry would bop swimmers on the head with volleyballs if their heads rose too high out of the water.

Guns of Navarone! In a war zone! There was dark humor in that. They could not stop laughing. (He's still laughing.)

Once a burly South African security specialist asked if he could bring his training dog—a sleek, muscular Rhodesian ridgeback—to attend swim practice with him. Jay was sorry to have to tell him that no pets were allowed in the pool.

Still they came. A new shuttle bus route was launched to more conveniently transport personnel from the little palace to the pool. Two or three dozen swimmers regularly attended each session, and now military swimmers started to show up. Some were young Marines looking for stroke refinements. Others were career military men and women in their thirties and forties who would soon be completing their service and wanted to take advantage of their hard-earned fitness by competing in triathlons in civilian life. Though his swimmers' stamina and abilities varied, Jay had pointers for them all. It began to dawn on him that as much as he liked swimming itself, it was the teaching he enjoyed most.

Jay ordered grab bags of equipment to outfit his swimmers: caps, goggles, kickboards. He'd always loved the creative tools and tricks that went along with teaching someone to swim—the ping-pong balls that you could blow across the water to encourage a relaxed, focused breathing rhythm, or the pull buoys that let you feel the tick-tock motion of your hips as they rotated in the water. "Some of the swimmers, like the security guards from Peru or Nepal, they were so poor—they lived a hard life and sent all of their money home," Jay says. "The fact that someone would give them a cap or a two-dollar pair of goggles meant a lot." He paid for the gear out of his own pocket.

THE SWIM TEAM as we know it in America has its roots in England, where swimming emerged as a collective sport in the early 1800s. Though a seaside culture had developed in the previous century, it centered mostly on bathing and swimming for hygiene and health, not for competition. The first municipal pool in England, the St. George's Baths, opened in Liverpool in 1828, and a slew of others followed.

Early swimming clubs began to form at private boarding schools, including Eton College; the school-age boys there kept records of group swimming adventures in Scottish lochs and English rivers. By the early 1840s, the college itself had a swimming requirement and kept a registry of those who did and did not pass the swimming test. Such a pioneer was Eton in English swimming that a few decades later the college's swimming teacher would publish an illustrated, gilt-edged handbook called *The Art of Swimming in the Eton Style*. The most significant swimming club of the era was the National Swimming Society, founded in London by a wine merchant named John Strachan. In the 1830s, the NSS hailed the salutary benefits of swimming, and organized races in the Serpentine and the Thames Rivers to inspire the public.

In one race, the prizes were silver cups and snuffboxes.

(How very English!) The NSS eventually gave out silver medals to other local swimming societies that were being formed at the time—in Oxford, in Glasgow—to use as prizes in their own races. Its members also provided free lessons, but only to the male public. It was not until 1859, with the advocacy of the influential writer and social essayist Harriet Martineau, that select hours and days were set aside for female swimmers at public swimming baths.

"English women have four limbs, and live in an island, and make voyages, and practice sea-bathing, and need exercise in the water at school and at home, and go out in boats—in short, run the universal risks in regard to water," Martineau wrote, with a somewhat wry tone, in an 1861 book of essays. Because of this, she asked, don't they have a claim to be taught to swim, just as men do? The girlhood struggle with physical modesty was no small thing in the Victorian era, and Martineau was concerned with the negative influence of gender on one's state of health. At the time, a few swimming schools were opening up in England for women, but Martineau had a firm universal prescription: swimming lessons for all children from a young age.

She'd observed girls learning to swim at a Parisian public bath moored in the Seine, all made possible with head-to-toe clothing, waist belts attached to a rope, and male (gasp!) instructors. She wanted the same opportunities for English girls. Martineau was up against more than a few stubborn taboos when it came to girls' swimming. Remember that the centuries-old practice of "swimming a witch," or throwing a suspected witch into water while bound—if she sank and drowned, she was innocent; if she floated, she was proved guilty—was not unheard-of in nineteenth-century England. But Martineau persisted. "In most countries in the world—actually over the greater part of the inhabited globe—the children swim as soon as they walk, if not earlier," Martineau observed. From Egypt to Mongolia to indigenous America and Polynesia, she wrote, "the human being is amphibious." There it is again: the ideal of amphibiousness, described as a desirable state for, well, everyone the world over.

In nineteenth-century England, though, swimming traditions were just getting started, as hundreds of clubs across the country took up the cause of promoting swimming. Some of these still exist today: the Serpentine Swimming Club (founded in 1864), the Otter Swimming Club (1869). The numbers of casual recreational swimmers increased as municipal pools opened all over England.

In August 1875, one of the world's first international swimming heroes emerged: Matthew Webb, a British steamship captain, made the first successful swimming crossing of the English Channel. The distance between England and France is twenty-one miles at its shortest, though Webb's zigzag course made it nearly double that. His genial, mustached face ended up on matchbooks. Eight years later, in Canada, Webb attempted to swim across the Niagara River at the foot of Niagara Falls and drowned in a whirlpool, but the fever had caught: by 1890, amateur swimming federations had formed in England, Germany, and France. Around the world, what began as fishing and foraging traditions and communal bathing customs evolved, in their own circuitous fashion, to formalized clubs where people could learn to swim. Mostly they were places to practice the sport, together.

Harriet Martineau, it would seem, had her way after all: when it comes to practice and participation, the most popular sport in England today is swimming. In my research into early swim lessons, I came across a vintage black-and-white photo taken in September 1906. It shows two tiny towheaded children suspended in the Thames River from what are essentially oversize wooden fishing poles tied with rope. The poles are held aloft by two male teachers, bent over and arms tensed, frozen by the camera mid-instruction. In the background, a flotilla of rowboats conveys fully clothed adults (parents? passersby?), all with hats and one with a parasol, in safe and distant observation of the lessons.

As I examined the scene, the only bit that resisted stillness— that seemed to me kinetic in some ineffable way—was the space occupied by an older, round-faced child who bobs in the water between the small children in the foreground and the boats in the background. That child, I thought, is the end result of these lessons and labors, on full display. Grinning, untethered, and swimming free.

EVERY YEAR, 372,000 people die from drowning. That's more than forty people every hour, every day. In 2014, the World Health Organization released a global report on drowning to launch the first worldwide strategic prevention effort. Their goal: to target drowning as a public health challenge.

Just because you know how to swim, of course, doesn't mean you won't drown. There are all kinds of factors that contribute to drowning incidents; for example, there is some research that shows parents are less attentive to their young children in water when those children have had swim instruction. But the vast majority of drownings happen in low- and middle-income countries where people have close, daily contact with water—among fishermen, say, or farmers ferrying their goods by river or children fetching water from a well or pond. Even in places with a strong swimming lineage, swim instruction is lacking. In Thailand, for example, where the encroachment of modern life has severely eroded the ability of Moken sea nomads to continue their centuries-old nomadic diving and fishing traditions, the World Health Organization in recent years has had to establish structured swimming programs to boost swimming skills in younger generations.

Similarly, in Madagascar, an island nation off the southeast coast of Africa, swimming is a luxury. Andry Rambolamanana's family did not have money. But when Andry was a boy, his aunt asked his mother if she could bring him to a swimming course held at a private Catholic school. At the class, the instructor lined all the children up at the side of the pool. Then he told them, one by one, to jump in.

"I will never forget him," Andry tells me. "Because the experience was horrible! Our first time! To jump! We did not know how to swim at all. But the teacher told us that if we did not do it, he would come for us." Trembling and near tears, six-year-old Andry stood at the edge, unable to will himself to get in the water. The instructor came up, grabbed him, and jumped in while clutching Andry. There was a whirl of bubbles and tears and terror. Andry doesn't remember much after that. "I don't even know how I got out of the water," he says, "but I did not get back in."

Andry the shivering child grew into Andry the big, athletic man. With massive shoulders and curly dark hair, Andry cuts an imposing physical presence. When we video chat—he is in Paris, where he now lives, and I am in San Francisco—he fills the frame with his bubbly cheer and wide grin. As he shares the story of his first experience with water, though, he seems to shrink into himself, retreating somewhere in his memory. But it is critical backstory to his experience in Baghdad—the best way he can tell me about swimming is to describe what it was to him since he was a child: a scary thing.

He was gifted on land. At university in Antananarivo, the capital of Madagascar, Andry was fond of all sports; in addition to being a kickboxer, he played basketball and took classes with a friend who was a taekwondo master. On Wednesday afternoons, the university offered students free use of its athletic facilities, and that's when Andry reacquainted himself with his old nemesis—the pool.

After so many years, he told himself sternly, I must learn swimming. Andry began going to the pool, without instruction, doing his own thing, splashing like crazy. After some days or weeks of patient trial-and-error, he was able to go the whole length of the pool. "But it was very exhausting, because I'm making all my effort to get movement!" he tells me, eyes wide. His shoulders quake; he pantomimes his flailing stroke and laughs, a deep, bass-toned *heh heh heh*, at himself.

That's precisely the level of swimming experience he brought to Baghdad when he arrived in late 2007, a few months before Jay did. When Andry laid eyes on Hussein's palace pool, he was dazzled. By that time, the army and security guys working in Baghdad were familiar with the opulence, and acted accordingly—meaning they thumbed their noses at it. They did cannonballs and strutted around. "They kind of felt like they owned the place," Andry says. But he had reverence. "For me, I couldn't believe it. *We can swim here?!*"

Andry first met Jay at work. As a sponsor for newcomers, he was the first to show Jay around the Green Zone, driving him back and forth in a golf cart. He was there by the trailers on Jay's third day, when Jay and J.P. got blown up. Every night, around nine or ten p.m., Andry tried to get to the pool. Jay would already be there, doing his laps. Andry would start his inelegant windmilling.

"I didn't know he was observing me," Andry says, "and then one evening he said, 'What the heck are you doing?'" He laughs at the memory. "I really just wanted to go to the end of the lane." Jay demonstrated the little things that he showed to all his beginning swimmers: Try blowing bubbles. Get comfortable with your head in the water. Practice floating while still, then floating with a small kick. Andry did as Jay said, and he felt the difference immediately. "It became easier, the flow was more natural," Andry says. "And that's how it started."

Little by little, Andry made improvements. He developed flexibility to go with his strength. For the first time, he could do a lap without being exhausted; with Jay coaxing him to keep going, he swam three more without even realizing it.

Andry learned all four competition strokes within six months. On his thirty-fourth birthday, he swam thirty-four lengths nonstop. Soon Jay had Andry coaching the military swimmers, too. Andry had his doubts: What am I going to do with these guys? They're so much better than I am. But he followed Jay's levelheaded example: he wrote up a plan of exercises for the advanced group, ran the swimmers through their drills, and observed them carefully. He tried to emulate Jay. As more swimmers came, Andry saw that Jay's real talent was in giving confidence to whoever showed up. There were people who had never been in the water. There were people who were afraid to put their faces in. There were people who couldn't complete a lap. All those kinds of fears could be conquered. This is how you do it. Play with the water. Blow bubbles. Be like Superman.

"And that's what I did," Andry tells me. "I passed along that knowledge."

One day both men were driving through the last checkpoint before the little palace when there was a direct hit on the United States Agency for International Development

(USAID) compound next door. The sirens went off, the big-voice "TAKE COVER" warnings blared, and the mortars started dropping, all terrifyingly close. Jay and Andry exited their cars and ran for cover. Andry managed to get inside but lost track of Jay. He began to panic. The resounding booms continued, but still he did not see Jay anywhere and could not reach him on the phone.

As soon as the attacks lessened in ferocity, Andry came tearing out of the building to look for Jay. He found his friend—one blast had sent Jay skittering down the lane into a cement wall, a little stunned, but in one piece—and dragged him inside.

As Andry talks about Jay and the time they shared in Baghdad, something snags in his voice. His eyes grow damp, his words deliberate. Coach Jay showed Andry Rambolamanana that the impossible was possible. "I never told him this," Andry says, "but I think of Coach Jay as my dad. He is my mentor in every way."

10

Chaos and Order

Most people came to Baghdad on one-year assignments—a swimmer might be with the team for a couple of months, say, before cycling out, but then someone else would join. Over the two years that Coach Jay was stationed in Baghdad, his swimming roster grew to more than two hundred people.

Certain swimmers stood out, like the irrepressible force of nature that was J. P. Santana. A lively, squarely built man with a defiant streak, J.P. lost the lower part of his right arm from grabbing a high-voltage power line as a teenager. Though he'd learned to swim as a child, he was left with burn scars all over his body. "I was shy about getting back in the pool after that—afraid, really," J.P. says. "I'd forgotten how to swim, so I was first in line when Jay opened the classes."

His right shoulder muscles, scarred and less flexible than his left, made him wonder if he could get back to swimming at all. "Once I hit the pool, I started to swim desperately, afraid I would go straight to the bottom," he remembers.

"What I learned with Jay is that I need to find that balance—in swimming and in life."

During the month of April in 2008—the "surge" in US military activity—the New Embassy Compound was not yet open. When things got hairy during a sustained period of shelling, the cultural affairs staff, including J.P. and Jay, had to sleep in the office, which provided more hard-shell protection than the flimsy, tin-can residence trailers. "We were without water for half a week, food was the same every day, and an Iraqi friend told me, 'Now you see how it is for the middle class in Iraq,'" J.P. remembers. "But we were lucky. Our only concerns were: don't get killed by a rocket, clean yourself with a handkerchief, and eat the same meal for a week." Compared to what the troops were facing in the field or Iraqis in their everyday lives, he adds, "We were blessed."

Being allowed back into their personal trailers was like being let out of prison. Being in the pool, then, felt like nothing short of exhilaration.

"Balance," J.P. had told me, "in swimming and life." The grim, weighty strictures of war make one long for a little levity. Jay himself was especially struck by the young soldiers who came in droves to the pool. Whether they were enlisted in official military service or under security contract, it was a different population of the world than he'd known in the past. "These were very hard young guys, accustomed to going on eighteen-hour missions," Jay says. They'd come back to Camp Victory—the home base for all those combat, urban-patrol, and sniper-detail Marines—smelling of cord-ite, and they'd prop their weapons up. "What do you think was their favorite, can't-miss TV program?" he asks me. "*Gilmore Girls*, of course."

After swim practice, the military swimmers would get back into uniform. In a complicated place that was so reliant on hierarchy and social order, Jay began to think hard about the way that swimming stripped people down to their bare elements. "You lose even more of your normal identity than if you got dressed for tennis, for example. You're just skin, cap, goggles," he says. "The outfits for swimming are at the bare minimum—their other identities aren't visible. With two military people, you can't tell who's the officer and who's the enlisted man."

That was a bigger deal than he'd realized. He thought in particular of the impoverished Peruvian guards, hired by the thousands to bring security and safety to American embassies and combat zones. "For them to shed that, and come learn swimming, just like the Americans and the other foreigners they guard day in and day out. To have that same privilege, it meant something."

Listening to Jay and Andry and J.P. gives me a sense of what swim lessons in international waters can do. "Nowhere else was there such a mingling of soldiers, diplomats, Iraqis, and other nationalities," Coach Jay says of the pool and his swimmers. Differences fell away in the water. Chaos turned to order. I remember what Kim told me about being stripped down to our essential selves in the water and how it allows us to see each other in the most basic way. In the far-flung land-scape of the embassy compound, the pool and the lessons in it had the focal power of a call to prayer. It was a way to recognize humanity, in a place of deep *in*humanity, through a kind of communion.

By the middle of Jay's stay in Baghdad, many Iraqis had stopped working in the Green Zone because it had become dangerous to be affiliated with the American military, USAID, or the embassy. Suspicion and misunderstanding came from every front. Were you a spy? Were you making a suspicious amount of money? Were you going to abandon Iraq and your family and traditions for America? There was, and continues to be, the problem of integration. But some Iraqi staff remained at USAID, and they rode the shuttle over to the pool to take swim lessons. Being in the pool was an opportunity to not get singled out for attention, be it positive or negative. They could swim, and learn, just like anyone else.

It was a profound thing, an altering of perspective, of possibility, of who you could be in the world. As I learn more about the Baghdad swimmers, I start noticing how the water is a privileged space and what an invitation to that space can mean for all kinds of tribes. I watch documentaries about transgender swimmers and autistic swimmers and how swimming pools mean freedom for their bodies, their minds. Entry into that water can feel like a restoration of power—"a serene power," one swimmer says, in the documentary *The Swimming Club*, about a transgender swimming group in London. And for autistic swimmers who finally have a team—the Jersey Hammerheads of Perth Amboy, New Jersey—that allows them to compete with everyone else, I see how swimming gives confidence through community.

As Jay sees it, his greatest achievement in Baghdad was providing his motley crew the rare opportunity to be together, all in the same pool. Not that there weren't issues. There was one man who spent his time with goggles on looking at women underwater, and several other men who came and sat at the edge of the pool, spectating, but Jay dispatched them firmly: "If you come, you have to swim. And we don't take kindly to oglers." (He had Andry's bulk, plus the looming presence of a couple of combat servicemen, to back him up.)

To organize the Baghdad swimmers and smooth their social frictions, Coach Jay drew on his experience as a swim instructor in Baltimore but also on his life's work as a cultural liaison in Africa and the Middle East. Talking about conflicts reminds Jay of his time serving in Cairo, when representatives of different countries struggled to get through Arab League meetings. There was one that ended in a food fight. "In Baghdad, at least nobody accused each other of peeing in the pool," he notes dryly, "even though they might have thought it."

IN ANDRY'S CASE, something that started out as play surprised him by becoming an essential escape hatch to somewhere else. "It's like reading books—when you're in it, you're not in the world outside," he tells me. For someone who had never before experienced war, being able to disappear was critical to his well-being.

"When people ask me about Madagascar, I tell them we don't know war," he says with a light laugh. "We don't know what that is. Even back in the time when the French came to take the country, we just gave it to them. It's a joke, but we honestly don't have that kind of feeling of conflict as much as other countries do."

In the world of wartime—unpredictable, unstable, and fickle—the pool, the lessons, and the team provided stabilizing ballast. Coach Jay left Baghdad in 2010, and Andry soon followed. "Someone from the military side tried to pick up the lessons, but he made it no fun, as I understand it," Jay says. The swimming lessons lasted a month or so after that and never began again. Today, the Baghdad Swim Team has scattered. Jay still works on cultural exchange programs and Middle East issues. He's busy building a boat in his garage, a thirteen-foot Jimmy Skiff with an outboard, nice for waters there and in Maine. He stills swims at his neighborhood pool, just three hundred yards from his house, outside Baltimore. Andry lives with his wife and toddler son in Paris, in the 15th arrondissement.

Recently Jay took his daughter, Lizzie, to France for a visit. They sought out the city's historic municipal pools, built in the 1930s. Andry still has a locker full of goggles and swimming equipment from Baghdad. Jay says that when Andry is ready, he will have all he needs to teach his little boy how to swim. And in Juarez, Mexico, J. P. Santana is still swimming two or three times a week. The pool is one of his best memories from a tough time. "To me, the swimming classes were like an accent of joy," he says. "We border people say *la cherry en el pastel*, the cherry on top of the cake. Or as an Iraqi friend would say: the lamb's head at the top of the biryani."

Not long ago, I zoomed around Baghdad using Google Earth and lingered on the bird's-eye views of the Republican Palace and its once-glorious pool, shaded by lush palm trees. It's drained of water now, as dry as the surrounding desert sand, but you can still see the shady perches along the edge of the pool where, once upon a time, a group of lonely swimmers paused for breath, and found each other.

COMPETITION

~

There is no passion in nature so demonically
impatient as that of him who, shuddering on the
edge of a precipice, thus meditates a plunge.

—EDGAR ALLAN POE, "The Imp of the Perverse"

I think of the salmon as the ultimate swimmer. "Salmon fry: five to ten weeks old and swimming." It's a caption I discovered on an illustration diagramming the salmon life cycle, and it unexpectedly moved me. Fish, of course, are born to swim. It's what they do. But there is a beautiful struggle in the life cycle of the salmon in particular, and a compelling analogy for the human struggle to swim at all. For the salmon, it starts as early as five weeks of age, the tiny fish still vulnerable as they wend their way downstream to the ocean. They are hiding under rocks and at the same time hunting for nymphs and insect larvae on which to feed.

The salmon life cycle is nothing short of miraculous, an elegant example of self-sufficiency and persistence—in other words, survival. A salmon begins life in a river, as a freshwater fish. Eventually, the fish smolts, changing its physiology to adapt to salt water, and swims out to the open ocean to spend its adult life. We don't know exactly where a salmon roams during the ocean phase; the different species of salmon in California distribute expansively over the North Pacific and the Bering Sea. But this is where a salmon grows, and explores, spending up to eight years in the open sea. And then it returns to the fresh water from which it came. It's easy to see why the aboriginal peoples along the northwest coast of North America hold the salmon in high regard in their mythology; in these cultures, the fish symbolizes instinct and determination, and renewal. Here, the salmon is also a primary food source. Here, the life cycle of the human is dependent upon the life cycle of the salmon.

When a salmon is ready to return to the freshwater river of its birth, it is transformed again. Depending on species and sex, it will grow a hump, or canine teeth, or it will develop a hooked nose—a bit like a prizefighter, in preparation for asserting its dominance. Some change color, from a pale silvery blue to a deep red. Eventually, the fish navigates its way back to the mouth of that very same natal river. Once it reaches fresh water, it stops eating. It becomes, by virtue of environment, something else, with the singular goal of muscling its way upstream to the place where it was born. Only the strongest and the fittest can make it to the upper reaches of that river, where it spawns and usually dies, leaving behind its body to enrich the waters. And so life begins again.

The salmon is a handy symbol for human aquatic strivings. For me, the story of swimming is also one of adaptation. We work to inhabit this element. Some of us also alter our bodies in pursuit of a goal. For most of us today—apart from the Guðlaugurs of the world, that is—survival as motivation, though, has given way to sport. Competition is how we can experience the adventure of assessing and moving through an attractive but decidedly inhospitable environment. It is only with sustained effort that we can master it.

FOR HUMAN SWIMMERS, what is competition? It's hard to know where to draw the lines around a contest for swimming supremacy, because we can define it in terms of all kinds of superlatives—longest, coldest, deepest, fastest.

Swimming is a useful skill with which to fish, yes, but also to fight. We can learn something of the nature of swimming competition from its origins as a wartime art. The ability was held in high regard in ancient civilizations from the Egyptians to the Greeks; to be ignorant of "either letters or swimming," Plato declared, was to lack a proper education. Herodotus described the Greeks as expert swimmers and thus able to make their escape to shore when their ships were destroyed in battle with the Persians (by contrast, he proclaimed, almost gleefully, "great numbers of the barbarians, from their ignorance of this art, were drowned").

Escape a sinking ship, cross a stream, flee your enemy: swimming's great value as a martial art since time immemorial is clear. Bas-relief artworks dating to 880 BC show an Assyrian king leading his army across a river with warriors swimming head up on what are thought to be inflated animal skins. In the Roman Empire, youth military training included bathing and swimming in the Tiber River. Julius Caesar was described, with much admiration, as a gifted waterman. In his biographical account of Caesar, the Greek historian

Plutarch wrote of the general at the battle of Alexandria, during the winter of 48 BC, escaping the Egyptians by leaping into the sea and swimming—belongings in one hand, stroking furiously with the other—to the shelter of a ship. Swimming would prove key in later military campaigns, as in the Roman conquest of Britain in AD 69.

What was once praised as a military art eventually became celebrated as an athletic art, performed in honor of the gods or ancestors and, finally, in pure contest for its own sake. In the same way that firing a pistol can be repurposed to signal the start of a race, the ferocious drive of battle could now be directed toward sporting competition.

Open-water swimmers like Kim Chambers, Lynne Cox, and Lewis Pugh can also serve as a kind of bridge, to help us understand how endurance and exploration in swimming can be reframed in the context of competition. There has never been a shortage of attempts to swim some tumultuous body of water—often resulting in death, or near to it.

One July morning in 2007, Pugh stood on the edge of the Arctic sea ice and thought of his mother. She was right. What he was about to do was not normal. Just as he was poised to become the first person to swim across the geographic North Pole, he froze. Not from cold—even though the subzero temperatures (-1.8 degrees Celsius, or 29 degrees Fahrenheit) would make it among the coldest waters any human had ever swum in—but from a creeping existential fear. *One shouldn't be able to swim at the North Pole in the first place*, he thought. Still he leapt, wearing just his Speedo.

In 2003, when Pugh quit his job as a maritime lawyer and set out to be a pioneer open-water swimmer, he had a vision of swimming down fjords and around wild capes and past icebergs where nobody else had ever dreamed of swimming before. "Like an aquatic Shackleton," he says with a laugh, one evening via video chat with me from his home in Cape Town, South Africa. "In my mind, it was a race between the three of us: me, Martin Strel, and Lynne Cox. They started before me and they took all the bloody warm stuff, so I was left with the cold stuff."

This, of course, is tongue-in-cheek: By the time Pugh started, Cox had been pushing the limits of human endurance and setting world records in cold-water swims around the world for decades. Cox tells me that she doesn't see herself as being in a race with anyone; her swims, she says, have always been about human ability and adventure. Despite her resistance to that portrayal, most of us are not immune to thinking about the world in terms of records, and the way we talk about open-water swimming achievements reflects this. Though Pugh himself claims that he doesn't compete in the traditional sense, he admits that he is a highly competitive person. In recent years, he has channeled those impulses in a different direction, using the superlatives that define an explorer—best, greatest, *first*—to his advantage.

"Being first is everything," Pugh tells me. By this he means that to win support for his cause, he must be first. Being the best, the first, in cold-water swims is a means to an end. It is his way to get people to pay attention, to give a sea-level view of our planet in climate crisis. The symbolism of the North Pole swim was clear: that he could swim across a place that you shouldn't be able to swim across, that used to be frozen. His 2015 swim in Antarctica's Ross Sea, in paralyzingly cold waters and severe wind chill, led to meetings with Russian ministers that helped remove the nation's remaining resistance to the establishment of the largest marine protected area in the world.

"For me," Pugh says, raising his eyebrows for emphasis, "it's a competition in creativity." He motions toward his dining room, where the table is covered with a sprawling, open atlas, its oversized pages spelling possibility to anyone who knows how to recognize it.

For most of us, though, competition is about speed. It's the chase, framed by a pool, in controlled conditions, with regulation attire. It is swimming competition the way it is conducted in the Olympics, for which the metric has always been the clock: how fast you can go.

~

11

The Splash and Dash

There is no faster event in Olympic swimming than the 50-meter freestyle. Its nickname is "the splash and dash." One length of the pool, on just the one breath with which you dive. Many world-class swimmers in this event don't take another breath in the twenty- to twenty-four-second duration, because it would slow them down. There's no time to overthink this race. The objective couldn't be simpler: get from one end of the pool to the other as fast as possible.

As a child, Dara Torres always had to be first, racing her siblings to the dinner table, to the car, to call their mother on her birthday. When Torres was forty-one years old, she had already retired from swimming three times. But those retirements didn't stick. Competition, she tells me by phone from her home in Massachusetts, is ingrained in her very being.

Her third swimming comeback brought her to her fifth Olympics, in Beijing, in 2008—the first American swimmer ever to compete in that many Games. At forty-one, she was the oldest Olympic swimmer in history. For context, one of her teammates in Beijing was Michael Phelps, who was twenty-three at the time. Torres won the first gold medal of her Olympic career in 1984, the year before Phelps was born.

But she wasn't in Beijing to set age records—she was there to win. Her extraordinary comeback brought her to the final of the 50-meter freestyle, for which she qualified with the fastest time, ahead of women less than half her age. Cate Campbell of Australia, who would go on to win the bronze medal in the event, was just sixteen years old. Torres's two-year-old daughter, Tessa, was home in Florida. *Someday, this is the race my daughter will watch to know who I am,* Torres thought. Thanks to her speedy qualifying time, she earned coveted placement in the final: lane four, one of the two middle lanes, with the best vantage point of her competitors on either side, and shielded by them from the slosh of the gutter.

In this sprintiest of sprint events, youth is an advantage. Fast-twitch muscle fibers, which supply the power—for the quick-response starting dive, the all-out, breathless controlled chaos of the arm stroke, the robust motor of the flutter kick, and the propulsive through-the-wall finish that's required to win—decrease rapidly past age twenty-five. (Slow-twitch muscle fibers, which govern endurance, stick around a little longer.) The current male and female world record holders in the 50-meter freestyle were twenty-two and twenty-three years old, respectively, when they set their records. It's a race where first and fourth are separated by mere hundredths of a second.

When it comes to swimming, the competition part has

always unnerved me. I don't like it all that much, and I still can't quite make sense of it, so I admit it's hard to write about. Thinking about racing makes me feel queasy. Even when I was a kid, contemplating a race would send me to the bathroom more than once during a single meet, my intestines in revolt. *Fight or flight!* I liked winning, and I liked swimming fast, but I couldn't figure out how to control all the other stuff that went along with getting your body into the revved-up state required to slay your rivals.

It's in the interest of understanding this inner drive that I seek out Dara Torres. Here is a woman so competitive that she floors it at the green light, she confesses to me, so other cars can't get in front of her. "I'm trying to be better with driving fast, since I have kids and all." Here is a woman so competitive that for the longest time she didn't care to swim unless she was winning. The nerves and the gut in revolt? An annoyance, surely, but a minor one on the way to being the best. "Getting to the top of your game, being there with the best swimmers in the world"—that is what she loved. She loved it so much she couldn't stay away.

I remember watching the television coverage of that 50-meter final in 2008; I went back to the footage before Torres and I talked. Torres waits behind the starting blocks, shrugging her broad shoulders and shaking out her long legs. She takes a deep breath and draws up her nearly six-foot frame, making a determined little wrinkle of her mouth. Her lean, muscled arms tense as she reaches up to adjust her black swim cap, printed with the American flag and "TORRES" in bold white letters. The crowd is cheering madly. She looks down the lane, focusing on its stillness, its clear, rectangular span of water, and cracks her knuckles.

Suddenly, she is calm. *I'm ready to go.*

IN THE FIRST modern Olympic Games, held in Athens in 1896 after being banned by the Roman emperor Theodosius I more than one and a half millennia before as pagan cult worship (the ancient Games were originally performed in honor of the gods of Olympus), there was swimming. Four events, four countries: Hungary, Greece, Austria, the United States. On a bright April morning, the swims were held in the brisk waters of the Bay of Zea, just southwest of Athens on the Piraeus peninsula. Twenty thousand spectators were in attendance, including the host country's monarch, King George I.

Participants were taken out into the bay by boat. Then they leaped off the vessel and swam furiously back to shore. Back then, "freestyle" simply meant that you could use whatever stroke you wanted. The United States, so dominant in other sporting disciplines, was shut out of the medal count; by one firsthand account, the American swimmers were "blissfully unaware" when it came to the realities of the icy Mediterranean Sea in spring until the crack of the starting pistol. For some, the shock of the cold water brought on a kind of momentary paralysis. The eighteen-year-old Hungarian swimmer Alfréd Hajós won both the 100-meter and 1,200-meter races. He later told reporters, "My will to live completely overcame my desire to win." (Perhaps his is a case in which survival and competition were conflated for a happy end.) There were no female competitors.

In 1908, the Federation Internationale de Natation, or FINA, was formed in London during the Olympics to regulate international competition in the sport, with eight founding nations behind it: Great Britain, Belgium, Denmark, Finland, France, Germany, Hungary, and Sweden. It still does that job. In Stockholm, four years after FINA's founding, women competed in aquatic events in the Olympics for the first time, though not American women.

In 1917, in New York City, a court stenographer named Charlotte "Eppie" Epstein founded the Women's Swimming Association, or WSA. She and a group of fellow secretaries and working women decided that swimming would be a good way to get exercise once they clocked out. In a time when women didn't perform strenuous activities or compete in sports, Epstein was a pioneer.

Though she wasn't herself an excellent swimmer, Epstein loved to swim, and she worked tirelessly to establish American women as a force in worldwide competition. The goal dovetailed with her work as a champion of women's rights. She was determined that women be taken seriously as athletes in sport. In one of her signature achievements as the "mother of women's swimming in America," as she was later dubbed, Epstein persuaded the US Amateur Athletic Union to endorse women's swimming in 1917—the only sport it recognized for female competition that year.

At the WSA, Epstein acquired the volunteer coaching

services of Louis Handley, an Italian-born Olympian who used the club as a lab to develop and refine the American crawl. The stroke was revolutionary at the time—it was a variation of the Australian crawl, but with a faster, six-beat flutter kick. Some form of the front crawl has been employed since ancient times, with appearances in Egyptian bas-reliefs from 2000 BC and, later, among far-flung indigenous peoples across North America, Brazil, and the Solomon Islands. It's now synonymous with freestyle by default—because of its superior speed, the front crawl is the stroke most people use in competition, if given the choice. Handley taught the American crawl to all the young women at the WSA— including a twelve-year-old named Gertrude Ederle.

The swimming costumes at the time were literally a drag: neck-to-toe black wool, which had to be covered with robes when swimmers weren't in the pool. Male swimwear was more progressive; the chief stipulation for men was that their bathing attire be distinguishable from underwear. In 1917, the American Association of Park Superintendents published bathing suit regulations that allowed men to wear tank suits, which consisted of shorts worn with a separate long shirt that covered the groin, for modesty's sake. But swimsuits for both genders were evolving rapidly, with less (and lighter-weight) fabric that gave more freedom of movement in the sport. Epstein eventually convinced the governing body to let female swimmers swim without stockings in competition—at the time, this was actually considered nudity—in the one-piece racing suit popularized by the Australian swimming champion Annette Kellerman.

Epstein was appointed team manager of the American women's swim team at the 1920 Olympics in Antwerp, and Handley assumed coaching duties. It was the first time American women swimmers were allowed to compete, and Epstein played a critical role in making that happen. WSA swimmer Ethelda Bleibtrey dominated at the Antwerp Games, winning gold in all three women's swimming events. Epstein and Handley would continue to work in partnership in subsequent Olympics, paving the way for—and training— Gertrude Ederle to become one of the best swimmers of all time.

Mindful of the example that was made of "Eppie's girls," especially given the risqué association in the public mind with women in bathing suits, Epstein carefully shepherded her swimmers to success both in and out of the water. She made sure they behaved as ladies, had impeccable manners, and dressed well.

Ederle was Epstein's ultimate success story: between 1921 and 1925, Ederle held an astounding twenty-nine national and world amateur swimming records—setting those records in an unprecedented range of distances and conditions, from sprints in a pool to miles-long open-water races—and became one of the era's most beloved sports heroes. As Glenn Stout notes in his biography of Ederle, *Young Woman and the Sea*, "'Ederle Sets World Record' became as common a headline in the sports pages as 'Ruth Hits Home Run.'"

During the 1924 Summer Olympics in Paris, Ederle won three medals, one gold and two bronze, despite adverse conditions: an injured knee and the fact that the women's team had to travel five to six hours a day just to practice in the Olympic competition pool. American officials didn't want the impressionable young women to mingle with Parisians of questionable morality—hence the exile to the outskirts of Paris.

Disappointed with her performance at the Olympics, Ederle set her sights on being the first woman to swim the English Channel. A swim crossing in the frigid, forbidding strait, often chopped by waves and wind, was considered a monumental physical feat during that era. In 1925, Ederle and Epstein traveled to England for Ederle's first attempt. She was disqualified when their British guide, thinking she was drowning, touched her halfway through the swim; a frustrated Ederle later said she was just resting. In the most epic of comebacks, Ederle returned the next year and smashed the men's record *by two hours*. Lloyd's of London took bets on Ederle, laying five-to-one odds against her making it across. Ederle's father, Henry, collected handsomely. She came home to New York and was greeted by a blizzard of ticker tape.

Charlotte Epstein eventually led her swimmers to more than fifty world records. Through the next decade and beyond, the *New York Times* wrote frequently about the Women's Swimming Association's "girl swim stars," whose monopoly on various swimming championships during the period was unparalleled. So many "local mermaids" had been turned out by the club that it was almost old news when a speedy new naiad was introduced in the paper's pages as a coming Ederle.

DARA TORRES FIRST broke the 50-meter-freestyle world record as a fourteen-year-old, back in 1982, the very picture of a speedy new naiad. She swam in the 1984 and 1988 Olympics, winning relay gold, silver, and bronze, and retired after college, thinking that was that. "At that point in my life, I was considered old," she says. She was barely in her twenties. But, like Ederle, Torres wasn't totally happy with her performance at those early Olympics. She hadn't yet won an individual medal.

Looking to get into television, she took a menial job as an intern at NBC Sports. One day, she was logging tape—the venerable figure skater Brian Boitano was talking about making a comeback, and what it would mean to him to do it. A bell went off in her head. *I want to do that.* Eleven months before the 1992 US Olympic trials, she moved to Florida to train.

Torres was elected a team captain of the 1992 delegation to Barcelona and won another relay gold. "I was the oldest woman on the team, at twenty-five," she remembers. "They called me Granny." She retired again and didn't get in the pool for seven years.

In the spring of 1999, at the coaxing of her friends and her mother, she unretired for the second time, training for the Sydney Olympics in 2000 and winning five medals, three of them individual this time. When she was walking out of the arena after her final event, a reporter stopped her for an interview. "You didn't swim for seven years before this," he said. "Do you think you'll be back at forty-one?"

"I was like, 'Yeah, right,'" she says. She went home and retired a third time, at thirty-three, thinking that she had nothing left to prove.

That reporter showed himself to be prescient. In 2008, at forty-one, nearly two and a half decades after her first Olympic medal, Torres was back in the pool. She took up swimming during pregnancy, in an attempt to get exercise while coping with nausea, and despite her burgeoning belly and the near-constant urge to throw up, she found herself unable to resist racing the middle-aged man in the next lane. It drove her crazy not to beat him. And that's when she began to suspect she was ready for yet another comeback. But it happened more quickly than she expected: a few months after her daughter was born, she surprised herself by swimming well enough to qualify for the 2008 US Olympic trials.

Competition kept coaxing her back to the edge of the precipice, as Edgar Allan Poe called it. This time, the precipice was lane four.

Lane four. We're back with Torres at the starting blocks of that 50-meter freestyle final in Beijing. The swimmers step up, shaking out limbs one more time as they listen for the race official's voice. *Swimmers take your mark*. At the beep, they fly off the blocks, with a mid-air undulation that propels each of them into the pool.

True to its splash-and-dash nickname, the 50-meter free is a frantic, foamy blur—in this case, it's one that lasts twenty-four seconds. In basketball, that interval is the shot clock. An NFL player can run the length of the field for a touchdown, with an eternity left over to do a funny dance. The international space station can travel a hundred and twenty miles. Twenty-four seconds is time enough to eat a doughnut, heat up coffee that's gone cold, compose a birthday text to a friend. But in the pool all you see is eight lanes of a barely contained tempest churning up bubbles from one end to the other.

In that race in Beijing, Torres held the lead from the start, her powerful arms turning over at a relatively controlled and efficient stroke rate. In the final push, her fingertips appeared to be the first to reach for the wall. In the slowed-down underwater footage, though, lane three, Britta Steffen of Germany, comes in strong on Torres's left. As Torres glides in, Steffen's hand surges just past, 24.06 seconds. Torres's time: 24.07 seconds. Steffen won gold by one-hundredth of a second.

One-hundredth of a second. It's less than a flap of a hummingbird's wing. Less than the blink of an eye.

Torres remembers being in the pool, dumbstruck. No matter the result, she wanted to be respectful, so she ducked under the lane lines to congratulate Steffen on the gold and Campbell on the bronze. As she went underwater, though, expletives and questions rattled around in her head. *One-hundredth of a second? What did I do? I'm going to be thinking about this for the rest of my life. How could I have done this better? One-hundredth?*

She called her personal coach, Michael Lohberg, who was watching from a hospital bed in Maryland, where he was receiving treatment for a blood disorder, and asked him what she did wrong. "You didn't touch the pad hard enough," he said. Two minutes after picking up her silver at the 50-meter medal ceremony, she was back on deck again to swim the anchor freestyle leg of the 4 x 100-meter medley relay. In that race, she swam the fastest 100-meter freestyle split in relay history. She hit the touchpad on the finish so hard that she tore a ligament and broke her thumb. They won silver.

More than she likes to win, Torres hates to lose. I ask her how she recovered from the one-hundredth-of-a-second heartbreak. "It did stay with me for a while," she admits thoughtfully. "I had to come to terms with it, after going over it so many times in my head, that the race was a perfect race for me. I had to be OK with it. I was mature enough, at forty-one, to not dwell on one-hundredth of a second." She realized she could lose a race and still have it be a perfect swim.

~

12

How to Swim Like an Assassin

In the sporting world, swim meets are a hybrid: individual events scored as team competition. Which means that though you contribute to your team's victory or defeat, the experience of a race is a lonely one. Even in a relay event, your particular sliver of team competition is conducted in solitude.

Hit the water, and all the sound and fury of the crowd is stripped away. You are swimming in a kind of sensory isolation, peripheral vision limited by your goggles, or perhaps by the glare of the sun. In your haste to get to the other end of the pool and back (and hand off to the next swimmer if it's a relay race), there is first and foremost your own brain to contend with. A track or cycling or gymnastics meet is similar in format, everyone ostensibly working in symphony, but the swim meet's aquatic environment enhances the athlete's solo to the extreme.

The view from within is what I'm after. What frame of mind does a competitor need to succeed at the highest level of this sport? I call up Jim Bauman, a sports psychologist who worked with the US Olympic swim team over four Olympic cycles, from 2004 to 2016, for a peek inside the elite swimming brain. A lot of sports psychologists describe swimming as 90 percent mental, but in a way Bauman thinks it's the opposite. "They talk about mindfulness, but I think of it more like mind*less*ness," he explains. His job, as he sees it, is to make that mental piece smaller and smaller and smaller, so that when it's time for the swimmers to race, "the 767 is on autopilot"—they're controlled by their biomechanics and their race plan, not their emotions or worries. The mental and emotional baggage is, as the flight attendants say, safely stowed away.

Every day, day after day, in the same pool. You can see people in the next lane, but you can't really talk to them. Back and forth, back and forth, staring down at the black line at the bottom of the pool. It's a lot of time to think, and if you aren't careful, fear can take over. Among elite swimmers, that line is a menace, a thing you can grow to hate. You show up on competition day and ask yourself, *Was all of that worth it?* Even if you're successful, Bauman says, the cavernous space of your head amplifies the ego and the self-talk and makes it all echo.

The best swimmer in the world at the moment, Katie Ledecky, may have a special knack for clearing her head. Fear is a major issue for most athletes, but Bauman thinks she's wired differently. Ledecky currently holds the world records in the 400-, 800-, and 1,500-meter freestyle. At the 2016 Olympics in Rio de Janeiro, she obliterated her own world records in the 400-meter and 800-meter freestyle races by jaw-dropping margins. In 2018, she beat her 1,500-meter record by *five seconds*. By the time she was twenty-one years old, she had set fourteen world records. By the time you read this, she may have added even more.

If you listen to Ledecky talk about swimming, you begin to realize how single-minded her focus is. Years ago, as a fifteen-year-old upstart preparing for her first international meet, the 2012 London Olympics, she visualized her race. She never visualized winning anything but gold.

"She was the youngest on that Olympic team, racing against the reigning champion in that champion's home pool," Ledecky's coach for four years, Bruce Gemmell, tells me by phone from Maryland, where he coaches the Nation's Capital Swim Club. That's where he trained Ledecky after London and up through the Rio Olympics. "When asked if she was nervous, she said she never let herself picture anything else but winning." He has a favorite way to describe Ledecky's mindset in competition. "She's not afraid of failure," he says, "but failure is never an option."

On a day-to-day level in practice as they prepared for Rio, Gemmell says she failed spectacularly—and that, too, was key. "She was always willing to stick her neck out in training, and she failed more than anyone else I've ever coached, but that's only because we set the bar so high," he explains. "She reached for it, and even if she didn't achieve the times on the sets, or if she faltered and faded, she succeeded in the attempts. And she came back the next day and did it again."

As an undergraduate at Stanford University, Ledecky is now a psychology major. For one course, How Beliefs Create Reality, she was asked to talk about how she had used goal setting and mental imagery to win her gold medals. In one PowerPoint presentation, she talked about Gemmell and explained how failure is a critical stepping-stone for success— and how not being afraid to fail helped her to believe that she could accomplish the goals she set.

Gemmell tells me that, in competition, Ledecky has a specific kind of confidence. It's not an arrogance. "Michael Phelps took that same confidence into competition," he says. "And yet at the same time, in the prep, Katie would be obsessed with any detail, or major thing, that she could in practice do to get better."

Bauman, the sports psychologist, has worked with Navy SEALs for years. He has even taken Olympic athletes to do obstacle-course training sessions with them in California. "People always ask me how Navy SEALs are able to maintain focus in such crazy situations, when so many things can be coming at you," he says. "What SEALs are good at is being able to find what is relevant in a situation, and they don't get distracted by all the irrelevant stuff, the noise. They focus on the job, the objective, and that's it."

Irrelevant stuff for a swimmer: *What lane did I get? Who's swimming next to me? Who's in the crowd? Where's the clock? What did social media say about me? What's the temperature of the water?* "That has nothing to do with your job as a swimmer," Bauman says. In training, you focus on biomechanics:

your start, your kick, your breathing and rhythm. He tries to teach his swimmers to do the same thing in a race. "Your job is to swim as fast as possible from point A to point B. What your competitor is doing is irrelevant to what you need to do. And that's the way the Navy SEALs think."

Athletes who can perform on demand—Torres, Phelps, Ledecky—are enough like SEALs that this was Bauman's mantra for the American swimmers in Rio, in 2016: *Swim like a dolphin, think like a SEAL.* "Clearly, the stakes are much different between elite athletes and special operations war fighters," he tells me, "but the thinking is similar." In the pool, Ledecky has been described as "an assassin," "stone-cold," "pitiless." When it comes to the best minds for swimming, I suppose it shouldn't be surprising that the most elite competitive swimmers share traits with the most elite fighters.

What sets Torres, Ledecky, and Phelps apart as successes includes the ability to grind it out, forever and ever and ever, in the interest of achieving autopilot—the mindlessness that Bauman describes. The constant rehearsal, and the unwavering focus that's required, is its own kind of endurance.

Phelps, the winningest Olympian of them all, did plenty of mental rehearsals for his Olympic victories. What a race looks like, feels like, smells like. What you want to happen in that race, in the form of a vivid script and images. What distractions may come and how to manage them. He visualized staying in his lane. "Stay in your lane" meant stop worrying about what everyone else was doing.

His longtime coach, Bob Bowman, told him not to say the word *can't*. Bowman did that, Phelps said recently, "so I could broaden my mind and believe that I could do whatever I wanted to." That, he thinks, was key to their success together.

But I can't help but point out that hyperfocus is hard to sustain over decades of swimming. Water erodes even the hardest rocks over time. At the elite level, a swimmer is in the pool twice a day, logging six to twelve miles a session, with precious few days off. It is a punishing regimen to sustain. The clock ticks. Lap after lap, the unchanging scenery. Over the years, even the steel-willed champion who ended up with twenty-eight Olympic medals broke down. The black line bedeviled him. In the chase for those medals, Phelps battled suicidal thoughts and depression. Competitive swimming is lonely. As time went on, the pool contracted, becoming a fishbowl he couldn't escape.

We can't really get inside the heads of elite swimmers, of course. We only know what they tell us. Like Torres, Phelps had temporary retirements. He became vocal about depression and mental health. He ended up in rehab in 2014, to deal with his substance abuse. In recovery, he tried to understand how the constant churn of competition wore him down and how he had questioned his own value as a person apart from the swimmer who won medals. He remembered that he loved to swim. That he still wanted to do it. But he realized that his personal objectives had shifted, from being a competitive swimmer first to being a husband and father first.

Post-rehab, in the lead-up to Rio—where he would win six medals, five of them gold—he spent most of his training time in an outdoor pool, which was new to him. For the first time, there was something else to look at. "You have a different energy outside," Phelps told *Sports Illustrated*. "You finish swimming and look up, and it's a blue sky with no clouds. That's pretty amazing to me."

An unofficial survey of popular swim team names, their native animal traits, and where they are found in the United States:

Barracudas: normally distributed widely in temperate, tropical seas; noted for large teeth, vicious behavior, and indiscriminate killing. Swim team sightings in California, Florida, Maryland.

Crocodiles: native to every continent except Antarctica and Europe; certain species have loud roars and powerful tails excellent for swimming. Significant swim team populations located in California, Indiana, Florida, and Texas.

Hammerheads: found in all tropical waters worldwide; male and female great hammerheads are both solitary and dangerous to humans, while scalloped hammerhead females tend to congregate in large schools. Swim teams widely distributed, from New Jersey, Maryland, and Georgia to California and Oregon.

Orcas: found in all oceans of the world, from the Arctic to the Antarctic; they are highly social, and whales in a pod swim together and coordinate their activities, including teaching younger pod members how to hunt and how to be good parents. Swim team populations have similarly wide-ranging communities, including locations in Georgia, Illinois, and Texas.

Sea otters: populating offshore kelp forests along the Pacific coasts of Russia, the Aleutian Islands, Canada, Alaska, Oregon, and California; can swim up to nine kilometers an hour underwater and are superb divers. Heavy overlap in swim team distribution, especially in California, but ranging to places including Wisconsin.

Terrapins: mostly used to refer to the diamondback terrapin, a species of turtle that lives along the eastern coast of the United States and is also abundant in the Gulf Coast; they spend roughly equal time on land and in brackish, swampy water, though they need fresh water to drink. They are quick to flee and are very good swimmers. Swim teams prevalent in California, Texas, New York, and Maryland.

What's a team mascot, anyway, but a spirit animal for that team? In these zoological naming conventions, we can read our ambitions as a species. We wish to be native swimmers, and merciless competitors. In the wild, speed, power, endurance, and cunning are prized, critical to an animal's success. And so it is in the pool.

13

Sharks and Minnows

From where I live in Northern California, it's less than two miles to the Albany Aquatic Center, where, starting around four in the afternoon, you can observe the life cycle of a young swimmer. In the indoor pool, where the warm water serves as an incubator, the youngest children get in first, their squishy, unmuscled limbs moving in whatever the opposite of coordination is, a sort of octopus-like profusion-confusion of arms and legs churning up foamy water as they convey themselves from the edge of the pool to its middle depths. Sometimes their forward progress slows to such a point that it appears that maybe, just maybe, they are moving *backward*, through some improbable loophole in the laws of physics.

These are the tadpoles and the sea horses. Or so they are called by their swimming instructor, a chirpy, bespectacled young woman who, despite the uniformity and distortion that latex swim caps and tinted goggles impose on the tiny faces of her students, somehow knows the names of every single one of them.

Thirty minutes in, the alligators and crocodiles enter the water, followed by the sea turtles and dolphins. I love the names of these groups; they indicate a ruthlessness on the one hand and a sweetly aspirational quality on the other. But somehow they all feel true. The older swimmers are learning backstroke; they attempt elementary dives in the deep end; they perform the underwater undulations that begin to approximate a recognizable dolphin kick.

An hour in, the thoroughbreds arrive. Here are the high school swimmers, broad-shouldered Aphrodites and Adonises all, with their unmarred, smoothly muscled physiques, their sturdy bodies as yet to be marked in any obvious way by life. This is what a swim team looks like, or at least the one here in Northern California. The boys wear Speedo briefs or body-hugging knee-length trunks; the girls have strappy one- and two-piece suits in all manner of color and coverage. They move confidently, in great loping strides, without the self-consciousness so common in kids their age, past the steamy heat of the indoor pool and into the bracing open air of the outdoor pool deck. They get in the water and they are of the water. They are creatures who belong there; they glide and ripple and move in harmony. They work, but it doesn't look like work.

It can take a long time to see if someone is going to be a good swimmer, to the tune of years, really. Press rewind on every Olympic swimmer—Katie Ledecky, too—and each starts out as one of those squishy little swimmers. There's home video evidence of Ledecky as a six-year-old churning away in the pool in her first race, periodically popping her head up and craning around to seek out visuals of her competitors. The final lunge for the wall, then her beaming face afterward. "What were you thinking about in the pool?" she's asked. "Nothing!" she exclaims, cheerily, crooked teeth everywhere. "Just trying *hard*!"

Many of us have joined a swim team at one time or another, and there is a shared foundational experience here that's worth examining. Battle past the desperate life-or-death phase of swimming, and you begin to appreciate how good the water feels. Join a team, and you begin to appreciate the company you keep. Competition happens when you get good enough at swimming to want to be better.

Right from the start, it becomes about speed, and technique. You work to refine your strokes, over and over again, to achieve—what? The win, yes, but that's fleeting, especially at this stage. Parse out the win for even the youngest swimmers and you realize that it's the rare coming together of effort and timing that lifts you for days. That's a feeling that any swim team swimmer knows, no matter their level.

Even now, I can trace a certain kind of physical confidence that I have all the way back to swim team. I am not a big person: five feet five on the days I remember to stand up straight. But the water is the one place I feel powerful.

I STILL HAVE in my possession a sheaf of pen-and-crayon drawings, carefully stapled together and dated July 4, 1984. In those pages—"From When I Was Six Years Old"—I stand on the diving board, glorious in stripes, before springing boldly into the air. There were so many ways to enter the water and swim for the ladder: forward dive, back dive, cannonball, can opener, pencil drop . . . I documented them all. It was summer. I loved swimming. That was the short of it.

The pictures show a joy and a practiced ease. But the operative word here is *practiced*. If you could peek at the pages *between* those pages, you would find a dense backstory. I could be free and confident and strong in the water because I'd already spent hundreds of hours learning how to swim.

We learned front floats and back floats: the calm suspension of our bodies in water. We learned to hold our breath and kick our feet: the foundation rhythms of propulsion. We learned elementary backstroke (up, out, together) and sidestroke (pick the apple and put it in the basket): the essential strokes of rest. We learned freestyle and how to breathe with our faces to the side: the drive of forward momentum. We learned breaststroke and how to breathe with our heads up: the safe sighting of a destination. All of this was drilled into us by repetition, every summer weekday, from nine to ten-thirty in the morning. We put in effort, then, to be effortless.

Our swim team was the Freeport Sea Devils. I loved all the different ways of getting faster: bobbing along with pull buoys, learning how to soar off the starting blocks, kicking until your legs burned. Most of the time, the payoff wasn't clear right away. My brother and cousins and I played games with the big kids: sharks and minnows, water polo, Marco Polo. Hook and ladder, in which one partner would hold on to the other's legs to form a single Frankenswimmer: one person kicking, the other pulling, inevitably resulting in a comically jerky push-pull action from one end of the pool to the other.

We swam year-round. In the summer, morning practices were held in the Olympic-size outdoor pool, after which Andy and I would come home and watch cartoons. In the winter, when practices were held indoors after school and ran late into the evenings, my hair would freeze on the car ride home.

We had pasta parties before big meets, to carbo-load our hungry, growing bodies. Aluminum-foil trays of lasagna, spaghetti and meatballs, baked ziti, made lovingly by team parents. Year after year at the division championships, we came in second to Echo Park, our rival team. One year, our coach made a deal with us: if we went undefeated in the season and beat Echo Park at the championship meet, we could shave his head.

That year, we won. We threw him into the pool and shaved his curly brown locks at the celebration party afterward. There's a photo from that night, our whole swim team swarming the pool deck. Little kids up front, arms raised in ecstasy, older kids cheering while perched up and down the ladders to the diving boards. There I am, sitting on the three-meter high-dive, helping to unfurl Freeport's bright red, white, and black team banner in victory.

The soundtrack to practice was the swishing echo chamber of the indoor pool deck, muffled in the water, the yelled instructions that only became clearly audible when we lifted our heads up to breathe or when we reached the wall at the end of a grueling set. Chlorine became my skin's default scent. During the high school season, I walked into home-room after predawn practice with goggle marks fading from around my eyes. To my classmates, it was the only evidence of my swimming life, other than the occasional swim meet results that came filtered through the garbled fuzz of morning announcements.

I END UP joining a swim team again around the same time my own six-year-old does. I spent a decade of my childhood competing, but it's the first time in more than two decades that I've trained and raced with others in practice. As an adult, I want to remember what it was all for. At the point of this comeback, I've just turned forty, so I guess I aspire to be an Everywoman Dara Torres. My team is the Albany Armada; Felix's is the Berkeley Barracudas.

The Armada is a Masters team, which means that it's part of US Masters Swimming, the competitive swim team circuit for swimmers eighteen and up. Established in 1970, US Masters now has sixty-five thousand members around the country and one thousand five hundred teams and training groups, and it sanctions regional, national, and international meets. It doesn't matter if you're a twenty-two-year-old water rocket just off a college team or a novice swimmer over eighty—there's a spot for you. Some swimmers compete in meets, while others prioritize training as its own goal.

The head coach of the Albany Armada, Carol Nip, is a sun-burnished woman in her early sixties who wears bright-red lipstick and a big smile. Though I'd been swimming at the Albany pool for four years, I'd never swum with the Masters team. It wasn't for lack of Coach Carol's recruiting efforts—I see why she has won national awards for superlative coaching and community building—I just wasn't sure I was ready for someone to tell me what to do in the pool again. I'd spent the last twenty years focusing on how to swim for fun and exercise, to swim an hour-long workout without worrying too much about speed and without the stress of competition. Masters swimming intimidated me.

On our respective first days of practice, Felix and I both feel the same nervous butterflies quivering in our stomachs. Those time-worn social anxieties—*Will it be fun? Will I be able to keep up? Will everyone be better than me?*—are streaming on loop. As I walk out on the pool deck, I'm startled by the momentary feeling that I'm walking with the shadow of my girlhood self.

When I was a child, competition was a way to assert integrity and dominance and power where perhaps there was none. I can see that there's something warlike in this—inasmuch as I've ever cultivated conflict, this is the arena. But along with that adrenaline rush comes a fear, of putting myself out there, in public, against a clock, against other swimmers. I don't want to care what other people think, but I do.

When I look back on it, there was a kind of "Paradise Lost" moment in my early swimming life, when I first understood how competition could get you down. I was an eighth grader on the varsity team, swimming in my first big championship final. It was the evening of the annual high school county meet, and I was surprised and delighted to find myself in the final heat of the 100-yard breaststroke. There was an older girl I looked up to, a senior. We swam on the same club circuit; I equated her in my mind with "goddess." I was a long-shot contender in the outside lane. She had the fastest qualifying time and got that favored middle placement in lane four.

In the moments before the race, she came up to me behind the starting blocks. I smiled excitedly, happy to see her. But the smile quickly dropped off my face when I saw the look on hers: she had a sick-to-your-stomach anxiety that was, I now know, contagious.

"I'm so nervous," she said, clutching my arm. This was not the girl I knew, who was always smiling and kind but also projected a cool confidence. This was someone else—a someone who was desperately holding on to me like I was her life raft. "This is my last race in high school." And then she said something that startled me: "Please don't beat me."

We went on to swim the race, and she ended up winning after all. After the race she hugged me, back to her usual effervescent self as she went to celebrate with her teammates. I'm pretty sure I did try to win, although I can't say that her words didn't change me somehow. Something crept in that day, an understanding that when you become accustomed to winning, you become afraid of losing. Competition was not a totally happy thing, not even for an eighth grader—and the worry of it could drag down the free-flying feeling I'd come to associate with it.

AT PRACTICE WITH the Armada, I look at all of us in the water, flitting back and forth across the pool in our flashy, colorful suits—one thing that hasn't changed is that Speedos are still as gaudy as they ever were—and I see a school of flashing fish. After just a few weeks, I realize that I'd missed training with a team, the motivation of swimming together. I find that it's easier to make myself swim fast for someone else. Having teammates picks you up and pushes you along. In that school of fish, there's a shared consciousness and a shared purpose.

I go home after a particularly grueling midday practice, and when I rise from my desk, my left shoulder complains. Or else it's my right. Some days, I give age a concession and take an afternoon nap.

One morning, Coach Carol hands each of us a little notebook. Before she lets us get in the water, she makes us scribble down two goals for the next year. What do I write?

1. Do something that scares me.
2. Swim in a meet for the first time in twenty-plus years???

Later, after practice, Coach Carol stops me outside the pool. "The Pacific Masters short course championships is coming up," she says cheerfully. "I think you can be really competitive in your age group. Mark it on your calendar!"

At these words, my adrenaline spikes, a Pavlovian response I thought I'd outgrown. But I'm curious about competing again. I find myself thinking back on those Sea Devil days. Who was that girl who once thrilled at a race? And what version of my competitive self would show up at the meet?

Competition day glints like an outdoor pool, all dewy blue and sunshine. On the early morning drive over the Berkeley hills to the Soda Aquatic Center, I feel my stomach turning over. My left shoulder is still a little cranky from when I surfed two days ago. Just enough to remind me of my forty-to-forty-four age group. To offset the anxiety, I decided to swim two fast, fun events: the 50-meter breaststroke and the 100 IM, or individual medley—twenty-five yards each of butterfly, backstroke, breaststroke, and freestyle.

The pool at the Soda Aquatic Center is a thing of beauty: eighteen competition lanes that allow two heats to run concurrently, with nine lanes each. The pool is so big that there are two extra lanes in between, left empty as a buffer. A thin, translucent layer of fog hovers above the cerulean water, waiting to be burned off by a still-sleepy sun. Off to the left, behind a set of metal bleachers and a digital timing board, there's also a dedicated warm-up pool, open for use between races so we can stay loose.

Hundreds of swimmers are milling about, swathed in the shin-length hooded parkas that are particular to swim teams: bulky, fleece-lined nylon monstrosities in all colors, heavy on the reds and blacks and royal blues, trimmed with gold and black and white, embroidered with inscrutable acronyms. MEMO. TOC. EBAT. ALB. (I know that last one, at least, because it's us: Albany Armada.)

I still remember what to do. I shed my layers in a heap under our team's shade tent and snap on my cap and goggles, being careful not to poke a fingernail through the delicate yellow-and-navy latex of our team cap. After warm-ups, Coach Carol hands me a rubber band—a reminder to always be flexible. She also presses a blue ribbon into my hand. "You've won already," she says, grinning. "It's your first meet since high school!"

At the lane assignment for my first event, the 50-yard breaststroke, I take a long look around. I can't help noticing a swimmer in the eighty-to-eighty-four age group standing nearby, wearing a black cap, a red team parka, and matching bright lipstick, a serene look on her beautifully made-up face. I look at her, and something about her contented presence settles me.

The official calls my heat, and I step up to the starting blocks, at the precipice of that gorgeous, glorious, ginormous pool. *Swimmers, take your mark.* At the signal, I take the plunge.

The rush of water in my ears, a *phroom* like the ocean. That delicious silence underwater, strong pull, kick, *gliiiiiide*. The fragment of time is so full of possibility, I almost don't want to break the surface. When I do, I don't hear anything. Arms and legs are moving mechanically now, executing the breaststroke they've been practicing so faithfully. And yet my mind is moving a beat behind, not quite there with my body. It isn't until the second lap of the two-lap race that I wake up—suddenly, and with startling clarity—and everything clicks into focus. The last fifteen yards, a surging in my limbs, as if I've just remembered to hit the gas pedal.

Afterward, when I'm not cheering for my teammates, I drift around the pool deck with a foolish grin on my face. I still have another race, and the results won't come in until hours later. (I place third in both of my events.) I'm no Olympic swimmer. My goals are modest; the stakes are low. But however fleeting it is, I remember what it feels like. A momentary lightness, the feeling of having done my ever-elusive *best*.

IN PRACTICE, COACH Carol offers constant calibrations. Keep your head between your arms on the breaststroke. Press. Your head is popping straight up and it's stopping your forward movement. Your right arm keeps crossing over on backstroke. Try reaching for three o'clock. Keep your hands apart when you enter on the butterfly pull. Out here, shoulder width apart, not together. On freestyle, lengthen your right arm, elbow high. You are entering short.

I keep these in mind as I swim on my own outside of practice. Press. Reach. Head down. Fingertips dragging. It's a constant refinement, and I begin to realize that the physical repetition can be a kind of meditation that transcends the simple goal of winning a race. I've never really thought about swimming in this way, since the frenzy of head-to-head competition always eclipsed it. Still does. (Even at forty, there's nothing like the impending anxiety of a race to send me straight to the bathroom.) But there is a Zen practice to be found here, in the motions, in the pool, in the *Karate Kid* "wax-on, wax-off" repetition until it's right. It is swimming as self-improvement.

We practice starts, turns, streamlines. We get up on the blocks and rehearse relays. As I become more and more immersed in this kind of intent practice, I think about what intrigues me about swimming as a sport—that the adversary is not actually the other person, though that other person is *there*, swimming alongside you. What I mean by this is that swimming competition is not like fencing, or wrestling, where you outwit the other person. Like running, swimming has a basic, elemental feel. Your chief adversary is the clock and, in this case, the water that you've got to work with to beat it.

14

Ways of the Samurai

Picture a silent samurai, submerged to his shoulders in water, swimming across a river with speed and efficiency—all while wearing a full forty-five-pound suit of armor.

In Japan, a country of islands, writings dating back hundreds of years describe samurai swimming. In feudal times, different *ryu*, or schools of swimming, developed; samurai protecting each region and geography had their own ways of navigating the local waters with artful efficiency. Nearly every clan had a *ryu* during the feudal period, from 1603 to 1868, when swimming as a military art blossomed under the encouragement of the Tokugawa Shogunate.

The schools of different warrior groups came up with a diverse array of techniques for sneaking up on an enemy, floating for long periods, and fording fierce rivers. These classical Japanese swimming martial arts, or *Nihon eiho*, evolved to prize grace and elegance, with deliberate movements that reflected conditions such as ripples and waves, so that the body and the water could move harmoniously as one.

In 1898, Japan hosted its first modern swim competition, in the port city of Yokohama, one of the first parts of the country to be opened up to trade with the rest of the world. Yokohama, understandably, was the site of many foreign firsts for this once-isolated nation: the first English-language newspaper, the *Japan Herald*; the country's first and largest Chinatown; and this first international swim meet, between Japan and a combined team that included England, Australia, and the United States.

Using centuries-old samurai swimming strokes, the Japanese beat the foreigners in the 100-yard and 440-yard races. It's a challenge to find any English-language record of this historic sporting event, but I tracked down a 1935 book about the history of swimming in Japan. In it, I found a reference to the mysterious "Englishman named Arbin" who managed to win the third event, the 880-yard race. Why those particular distances were selected for the races, I cannot tell you.

But I can tell you that the Yokohama contest holds a special place in Japanese swimming history. More than a mere swim meet, it symbolized a larger, head-to-head measuring up of Eastern and Western traditions and philosophies. In the meet, the English used the trudgen—imagine a head-up alternating front arm stroke, but with a kind of sideways leg thrash with each stroke. The Brit John Arthur Trudgen picked it up from indigenous tribes as a boy growing up in Brazil and debuted the stroke in England in 1873; two years later, he won a local competition using it, in record-breaking time. The trudgen was hailed as a breakthrough.

But the Japanese had their own version of an overarm side stroke that was incredibly fast for the time. Their victories showed that swimmers using *Nihon eiho*—one of the eighteen martial arts of the samurai warrior class, including horsemanship, archery, fencing, and hand-to-hand combat—could compete and win against swimmers using Western techniques. The competition had an undercurrent of nationalist pride that coincided with the Meiji period and the modernization and unification of Japan.

In the early twentieth century, Japan began sending more swimmers to international swimming contests. During this period, strokes in the West were rapidly developing, and the Japanese worked hard to catch up. They adopted the latest versions of the front crawl stroke being employed by their competitors and studied techniques from books that they imported from England and America.

One modern pool was built in Osaka, at a middle school, and students there were taught the crawl stroke. It was at this middle school that a young man named Katsuo Takaishi began to swim competitively; in 1924, in Paris, he became the first Japanese swimmer to garner attention at the Olympics, managing fifth-place finishes in the 100-meter and 1,500-meter freestyle races, and a fourth-place finish in the 800-meter relay with three of his teammates. It was a rallying cry; the next year, all the disparate swimming groups in Japan were united under a formal amateur swimming federation.

Takaishi became Japan's freestyle swimming champion. In 1926, he and others were invited to a meet in Hawaii, where America's best swimmers were waiting to race them. There, Takaishi thrilled his countrymen by shattering Johnny Weissmuller's Olympic records in the 50-meter and 400-meter freestyle events. This was a big deal: At the time, Weissmuller was the famously handsome face of American swimming and one of the world's fastest swimmers, having just won two gold medals in the Paris Olympics, beating out the legendary Hawaiian swimmer and surfer Duke Kahanamoku. Four years earlier, Weissmuller had been the first to break the one-minute barrier in the 100-meter freestyle. (That he would later go on to play Tarzan in MGM's blockbuster films and become an international movie star of the era is also worthy of note.)

What about the other strokes? During this same period, Yoshiyuki Tsuruta became Japan's dominant breaststroker—at the 1928 Amsterdam Olympics, he became the first Japanese swimmer ever to win gold, in the 200-meter breaststroke. He was vocal about the influence of the classical Japanese swimming martial arts on breaststroke as we know it; he described it as a "speeded-up form" of *hira-oyogi*, a stroke developed by the Kankai *ryu* that was especially intended for swimming in the open sea over long distances. He saw value in the long tradition of Japanese training techniques in breaststroke and the skills it took to swim it well.

It was at the 1932 Los Angeles Olympics that Japan's champions finally broke out on the world stage with extraordinary dominance. With Takaishi as captain and also part of the coaching staff and Tsuruta leading the breaststroke contingent, the team's swimmers dazzled with their fitness and speed. They took home a total of twelve medals, *more than a third* of all the swimming medals that were handed out; they won gold in five of the six men's swimming events, sweeping the medal podium in the 100-meter backstroke and performing near-sweeps in three other events. Tsuruta won gold again in the 200-meter breaststroke, becoming the first Japanese swimmer to win back-to-back gold medals in the same event.

At those Games, Tsuruta saw hope for the reinvigoration of breaststroke's popularity—and pride in Japanese traditions—with his younger teammate Hideko Maehata, who won silver in the women's 200-meter breaststroke. She was the first Japanese woman ever to medal in the Olympics. Four years later, she'd win her gold. With Tsuruta, the Japanese began a reign of dominance in breaststroke that has lasted for nearly a century and produced an extensive cast of Olympic medalists.

I LIKE TO think that each of the different strokes has its own personality. Breaststroke is often thought of as the slow stroke, but it's my favorite. It requires a raised-head breath with every pull; it lacks the overt, churning power of freestyle and backstroke, and the flashy, splashy show that is butterfly. (Butterfly, strangely enough, evolved from breaststroke in the 1930s, when practitioners discovered that an out-of-the-water arm pull was faster than an in-the-water arm pull. A variation of the butterfly was used in breaststroke competition until 1952, when it was accepted by FINA as a separate stroke; at the 1956 Olympics, butterfly was finally swum as its own event.)

Concealed behind breaststroke's deliberate pacing is a quiet strength. It came naturally to my brother but not to me. As a kid, I worked hard to be good at breaststroke and, by extension, to acquire that quality that I associate with it. I had the propensity to hurry, and still do. But breaststroke won't let you be impatient; if you do, you lose the glide, and the entire mechanism for speed that's hidden in the stroke. Rush, and you go slower. It's the paradox of breaststroke. Ease up, though, and you stretch, like taffy. Cut the quick bobs, and you're pulled along, effortless, smooth as the hull of a boat cutting through early morning glass on a river. That frog kick, working without splash underneath the surface, is your secret propeller.

During practice, I used to draft behind my brother when I felt tired, using his wake to save energy. "Stop dragging off me," he'd say, but he'd smile to soften the words. In a breast-stroke race, the pacing is different; you must be thoughtful with timing, not hasty, or you get nowhere. In a modern world that is so obsessed with speed, it's a good reminder of what's possible when we slow down.

In an effort to be a better swimmer, I've been tinkering with the mechanics of my strokes with Coach Carol: lengthening my arms, keeping my head more streamlined, pressing my legs together. I attend my son's practices, where whole tidal waves of little kids churn back and forth across the

198 | BONNIE TSUI

pool. When Felix emerges from the water at the end of a session, lips blue and skinny shoulders shivering, he reminds me of my brother. I ask Felix how his swimming is coming along, and he informs me that he doesn't like the cold water. "What about racing?" I ask. I've seen the way he ratchets up the effort if someone inches up alongside him in the lane. "Don't you like going fast?"

He thinks for a minute. "I don't like it if someone *tells* me to do it," he says. "I like it if it's my choice." Now he reminds me of me. Self-discipline in the pursuit of self-betterment is hard at any age, especially when you're a child. But I'm older now. I have the feeling that I have something to learn from Japan's swimming martial art about what it means to be better—patience, for one, but also a longer, meticulously studied view on how our bodies can work in all kinds of water.

WHEN I FIND out that there are samurai swimming competitions being held today in Japan—now picture that silent samurai gliding across a 25-meter swimming pool—that attract swimmers from as far away as Poland and England, I make the trip to Tokyo to seek out the leading practitioners of *Nihon eiho*.

In a Japanese television report, a samurai lowers himself into a swimming pool. I watch closely as he demonstrates *katchu gozen oyogi*, full armor swimming. He moves smoothly on a sideways path across the pool, legs alternately circling.

The metal-pronged helmet atop his head stays dry. Despite the blanket of riveted leather scales weighing down his torso, he slides along, wraithlike. "The armor is very heavy," the young man says with a little smile, after he has dragged himself and his water-logged equipment out of the pool. "But I'm delighted I can swim." (The news report, lucky for me, is subtitled in English.)

Another swimmer, this one dressed in swimming trunks and a black cap with white stripes, demonstrates a different, more dynamic skill: *inatobi*, gray mullet jumping. From a still and submerged position, the swimmer surges vertically out of the water, arms whipping back and head thrust forward, exposed to his very lean (and very tan) waist. It is the fundamental method of jumping while swimming to disentangle oneself from seaweed or other debris, or to leap onto a boat.

Finally, the most fundamental of all moves: *tachi-oyogi*, standing swimming. The young competitor's face is relaxed, his eyes trained on the horizon. His head moves near imperceptibly, the water in front of him as still as glass. It's as if he is on a very slow treadmill hidden just below the surface of the water. His head and hair are completely dry. Different schools have different variations, but the basics are the same. That familiar egg-beater kick used today by synchronized swimmers and water-polo players to propel their upper bodies so powerfully out of the water? It bears a strong resemblance to the method described in detail in sixteenth-century master scrolls from the Kobori *ryu*, which specializes in techniques to free up the hands. The muted cycling of the legs is meant to be efficient and to keep the upper body stationary and stable. The version of the egg-beater kick used by the Japanese synchronized swimming team comes directly from the Nojima *ryu*.

I learn that if you're good at standing swimming, you can do anything in the water: write calligraphy, load and fire a rifle, duel with swords. You can carry weapons and flags. You can shoot a bow and arrow with great accuracy while nearly submerged. Remember that the feathers on an arrow need to be dry to fly true.

In the news segment, we see two men fight, each gripping his wooden sword with both hands. They shout and circle each other warily, as if they are dancing. But they're treading water, in a lake, far from shore. We see two women swimming *nukite*, the withdrawing hand style. This high-elbow, crawling arm technique is used to swim facing the wind and waves or when crossing the tide; it allows you to cut through the waves with your shoulder and avoid being overwhelmed by the foamy force of a breaking wave.

MIDORI ISHIBIKI IS a modern-day master in the age-old art of samurai swimming. Appointed by the Japan Swimming Federation, Midori is one of eight people who are responsible for preserving the swimming martial art of Japan. Like any other martial art—judo, say, or kendo—*Nihon eiho* is governed by various levels of practice, and each level requires years of training and exams to move up to the next.

Midori grew up in Tokyo and now lives in Kamakura, a seaside town an hour south of the city. Fifty years old, with reddish brown hair styled in a bob framing her round face, she can glide across a pool with barely a ripple. But *Nihon eiho* isn't just about physical skills: "It also emphasizes a spiritual path," she says in her perky, British-accented English, which comes from years of living in Norwich. "It's like meditation."

Old Japanese texts teach that swimming in freezing water cultivates perseverance; submergence leads to patience; diving fosters bravery. Floating of the body leads to serenity of the mind. The mastery of rescue and resuscitation is a sign of wholehearted benevolence.

Midori began studying classical swimming techniques with her master when she was thirteen, during summers at the beach in Chiba, across Tokyo Bay from the city of Tokyo. Her club's current master, Kazuo Yamaguchi, is now in his mid-eighties, and Midori still studies with him every summer. But these days the student is also a master, and while in Chiba she in turn instructs more than two hundred junior high students from their school's clubhouse. Theirs is the Suifu *ryu*, which devised practical ways to swim efficiently on the open sea and rivers—to safely get through waves, say, or to quickly retrieve something floating nearby.

Though samurai swimming is at the roots of Japan's swimming culture, its traditions are waning. But those tasked with its preservation see a direct line to modern Japanese swimming success in international competition. During an unseasonably balmy week in early May, I travel around

Tokyo to see what samurai swimming looks like today and what it means that people are still doing it.

My pursuit of Midori Ishibiki leads me to an indoor swimming club in Yokohama, where I am sweating profusely on the pool deck. The indoor pool deck is like a sauna turned up to the max. It causes me distress to be dressed in street clothes by the edge of a perfectly nice pool, but it's the only way I can take proper notes on the happenings in Midori's swim class. Today there are five *hanshi* masters—the highest level master there is in *Nihon eiho*—attending the class along with the regular students. One of the masters, Masaaki Imamura, the seventy-three-year-old vice chair of the Japan Swimming Federation's committee on *Nihon eiho*, is examining me curiously. He also thinks it's weird that I'm wearing street clothes.

"Why don't you swim?" he greets me with a deep, booming voice, as he issues forth a charming grin. "It is very hot." He is wearing a black Speedo and a black cloth swim cap with white piping and strings that tie under his chin. The black cap indicates seniority in the Shinden *ryu*; white caps are given to beginners, much like the white belt in other martial arts like judo or karate. The progression of colors, however, varies by *ryu*. I manage to smile back, then grimace, and I'm tempted to dash back into the locker room to shed my heavy cotton dress and leggings so I can get in that water, too. But I can't chance missing what happens next.

The fifteen men and women in Midori's class circle and bow. Then, one by one, they stride to the water and slip in, smoothly and soundlessly, like ducks to the surface of a lake. After a few laps, Imamura hops out and volunteers to be my de facto sports announcer. "Why do we swim?" rumbles Imamura, with another winning smile. "Well, that's very simple, you see." Like a professor, he steeples his hands, and then proceeds to tick off the following on his slender brown fingers:

For survival: "Japan, of course, is surrounded by water."
For religion: "In Shinto practices, *misogi*—the ritualistic cleaning of body and mind with water—is sacred."
For fighting: "The samurai, to protect feudal territory, developed regionally specific swimming schools."
For competition: "Disciplines include diving and racing, say, or synchronized swimming."
For strength of mind and body: "The topmost principle in *Nihon eiho* is mind and water, together."

This last principle, he says, can be explained as *mizu no kokoro*, or "mind like water." On the bench next to us, he traces a finger on its surface with water as he speaks, writing out the Japanese characters. "This is the most important thing. There are many reasons, but when you get older, you can appreciate the Zen part, the master part, the philosophy."

We pause to observe Midori as she swims by. She wears a

black cap with two white stripes that signify that she is the director of her group. As the rest of the class watches from the side of the pool, she demonstrates the *nukite* style, that withdrawing arm stroke I saw on Japanese television, the one intended to cut through incoming waves as one heads out to sea. Because she does this all with seeming effortlessness, and with a smile, her at-homeness in the water makes me think of a friendly porpoise at play.

"Midori-san, she is very good," Imamura says, approvingly. He comments on her smooth, elegant stroke and emphasizes the power of her propulsion. "You know Kitajima?" he asks, referring to the Japanese breaststroker Kosuke Kitajima— perhaps the greatest breaststroker of all time. Kitajima retired in 2016 after winning double gold in the men's 100- and 200-meter breaststroke in the 2004 Athens and the 2008 Beijing Olympics. "Kitajima swims breaststroke like *Nihon eiho*—because he has one powerful stroke and then floats: a long, long glide." The power of that one stroke, he explains, is critical—it shows a mastery of pacing and patience.

"You can go very fast using these techniques, but that is not what it is about," Imamura says. "Now, in modern Japan, *Nihon eiho* is for older people who know it is not about racing, or winning, the way it is for young people. We practice, practice, practice, and work very, very hard to get to that place of Zen. It is about strength of mind."

Like Midori, Imamura has been a senior figure in *Nihon eiho* circles for decades. He learned *Nihon eiho* as a child in school, first and foremost out of tradition. He continued the martial arts practice because he liked the meditative quality that came along with the physical movements. "It's like tai chi, but in water," he says. "That's a good comparison. In the concentration, you find a peace."

The class splits into groups of three, and each group sets off swimming across the pool in a triangle formation: head up, arms alternating in a front crawl stroke, legs frog kicking. Each person is fully aware of the others in the group, making minute adjustments so that the whole group moves in synchrony. Different swimmers have different strengths and weaknesses according to their bodies, Imamura explains. The three-swimmer formation is an exercise in awareness—of your own body and others', and of the ever-changing environment, too—and control. "You can't work against water; you have to work *with* water," Imamura says. As other long-time coastal cultures, like the Dutch, emphasize, here, again, is the idea of water as ally, not enemy. Knowing how to survive water is what allows us to see it as a friend.

After class, the masters delight me with an invitation to join them for beers in a small pub across the street from the pool. Midori, Imamura, and I crowd around a wooden table along with another master, Saki Kozuma, a dimpled young woman in her thirties who stood out from the rest of the class by virtue of her radiant youth. Then a trim, bespectacled man with neatly combed gray hair materializes at the corner of the table: Akinori Hino, the head of the national committee on *Nihon eiho* himself. (I recognize him from the Japanese news report I watched about *Nihon eiho*.) On this Sunday afternoon, because Midori informed him of my visit, he has taken the trouble to put on a jacket and tie to meet me.

With this eminent group of swimming masters gathered, I ask what allure *Nihon eiho* holds today. Why do people take classes in the swimming martial art instead of other swimming lessons? What are they looking for?

"It's very fun!" Imamura exclaims. Midori laughs.

"*Nihon eiho* is to make yourself better," she adds, after a moment. "Maybe it's health, or lifestyle. Or something for your mind. Every single person is at their own level, and it lets you choose your own purpose in the practice. What is your best purpose? It can be time, or speed, but it's not just that. It can also be that I want to be more beautiful in my stroke."

Hino nods sagely. "The patience, relaxation, and slowness of it is what I find interesting," he says. He pauses as the proprietress of the pub brings a tray of beers. A round of cheers and *kampai*, then we continue our conversation.

Kozuma, the young master, learned to swim in school when she was in kindergarten. School-age swim instruction is mandatory in Japan. She started *Nihon eiho* at her university. "I liked thinking about how to tread water, how to catch water, how to exercise for your mind, too, not just for body." She teaches *Nihon eiho* to high school and college kids at a university swim club in Tokyo.

"The water is the last place where people cannot text, call, or find me," she says with a giggle—in her efforts to develop the next generation, she finds that *Nihon eiho* has unexpected benefits.

TONY CUNDY IS a big guy—six feet five and over two hundred pounds. But when he's in the water practicing *Nihon eiho*, he's mostly hidden away to chin level. He gets a different view of the world there. Recently, on a trip to London, he swam in Hyde Park, swans and all. "When you're in the water, because you're not breaking the water or splashing, dragonflies will flit past you, boatmen will glide by," he tells me. "Your understanding of the world is at the waterline, not underneath." He pauses, considering. "Though a swan did attack me once."

Cundy is the only non-Japanese person ever to be certified to teach *Nihon eiho*. He lives in Tokyo and works as a top advertising executive, but he grew up swimming in Plymouth, a prominent English naval town. As a young man, he was proud of being an accomplished and speedy swimmer in the Olympian tradition. He moved to Tokyo in 1995 when he was twenty-two to study aikido. Five years later, he began to learn about *Nihon eiho*. "And everything I thought I knew about swimming," he says, "went out the window."

He remembers being in the pool with his swimming teacher for the first time, talking to him at length about the swimming martial arts tradition. His sensei was standing in front of him, arms folded, nodding his head. But he wasn't standing on the bottom of the pool—he was standing swimming, *tachi-oyogi*, the Japanese style of treading water. His upper body was so still that Cundy couldn't stop staring.

A teacher dropping to the bottom of a five-meter pool, walking across it, and then floating serenely back up. A practitioner treading water with arms aloft, holding a five-kilogram dumbbell, for more than an hour. His sensei firing arrows across the water to hit the centers of various targets. Suddenly, he saw, swimming was not about speed or distance but about becoming skilled enough to handle whatever water scenarios he might encounter out in the world. He learned to develop movement and momentum in new ways, through the hips and legs, with much less use of the arms. It was a revelation.

"My swimming was always, *Head down, thrash away, down, up, down, up, how many laps can I do?* I never noticed anything else," Cundy says. "Now my head is always up, and I breathe through my nose. I can see every wave, and I'm very aware of my surroundings." Speed is just one component of *Nihon eiho*, not the fundamental objective. For the most part, Cundy sees it as a way to experience his environment more keenly.

Cundy has competed in different *Nihon eiho* events, including the annual national competition in Japan. Only two events in that competition are races, one of which employs the stroke that those Yokohama swimmers used to beat the foreigners way back in 1898. The examinations and competitions range from those time trials and weight holding to demonstrations of flag waving and armored swimming.

I ask him, half-jokingly, if he feels ready for battle. "Crikey," he exclaims, thinking for a moment. Then he points out that some of the principles are similar to the combat and treading techniques used by Navy SEALs (clearly the SEALs embody a host of ideals, like the superior mental toughness that sports psychologist Jim Bauman spoke of). But for all of *Nihon eiho*'s physical challenges and athleticism, it's the degree of thought and refinement—"the same kind of refinement that has been applied to lacquering your bowl, for that matter"—that keeps him swimming.

THE IDEALS OF samurai swimming have a clear philosophical resonance today. In his book *How to Think About Exercise*, the philosopher Damon Young revives the ancient idea of exercise as something that takes into account one's whole humanity—and not just what he calls "the bodily machine." Young observes that the tendency to think in dualism—jocks vs. nerds, sporty vs. bookish—is a false divide when it comes to physical and mental exertions.

Swimming's benefit, he argues, has as much to do with intellectual enhancements as it does the achievements of the body. The ideal modern swimmer focuses on the whole experience rather than the perception of exercise as a "tune-up." Important, too, is the pride we feel in the well-exercised body. "The fuller sense of self we have," Young once told an interviewer, "the more responsibility we take for it."

Over time, swimming has shifted from mere mechanics and survival—a military skill, practiced by men—to achieve a more intangible significance: a form of recreation, a pleasure, something that can sharpen your spiritual as well as physical health. This idea of swimming for wellness, emotional resonance, whole personhood, rings true to me. The physical is intertwined with the psychological.

In Japan, Sawai Atsuhiro is a bestselling author who writes about mind and body unification principles that develop *ki*, or life energy. He has also written about his experiences of studying to be a master in *Nihon eiho*. The technique that impressed him most was *shusoku garami*, which allows someone to swim with both hands and feet bound together. There aren't many of us who will face the possibility of breaking out of an enemy prison, having to swim across the castle moat to escape, but there's a lesson here. "Astonished, I watch a man with hands and feet tied swim across a pool with a motion that is a cross between a swimming frog and an undulating eel. He is able to swim on his front or on his back, head first or feet first," Atsuhiro writes. "And my teacher surprised us by saying, 'You believe you swim with the arms and legs, but you're wrong. You can swim without them. Look at a fish. Real swimming is using the whole body.'"

In my mind, the salmon surfaces again, that elegant example of adaptation, tenacity, and stamina. We are not fish, but from them we continue to take inspiration. In this case, the fish reminds us that swimming can be something to engage your whole self. From the rigor of swimming competition comes a devotion to swimming as holistic self-betterment.

The emphasis moves from body alone to body and mind, together. Think of a stream flowing into a river, a river flowing into the sea.

These waters run together in a way that helps me to understand why I swim.

FLOW

～

Water is H_2O, hydrogen two parts, oxygen one,
but there is also a third thing, that makes it water
and nobody knows what it is.

—D. H. LAWRENCE, "The Third Thing"

I t's in the opening pages of *Moby-Dick*. "Yes, as every one knows," Ishmael declares, "meditation and water are wedded forever."

Here at the novel's beginning, Ishmael calls our attention to the crowds of dreamy water gazers gathered along the shores of Manhattan on a Sabbath afternoon. See all those people, leaning over ever so far. They prove him right: the ocean's liquid fingers have a way of transfixing us in thought. Ishmael points out that the ancient Persians call the sea holy, that the Greeks give it a powerful deity of its very own. A maiden voyage sings with a kind of "mystical vibration." But what exactly is the magic of water, and what does it do to us? It's a mystery.

When we peer into a lake, river, or ocean, we find that water encourages a particular kind of reverie. Perhaps its depths can enhance our consciousness even more if, instead of just looking, we get in and swim.

We jump into that water and find ourselves in a curious

liminal space. Here we are, suspended, yet moving; floating, yet ever in danger of sinking. And if we swim with the current, instead of fighting against it, we find a momentary state, one of motion and yet paradoxical stillness that is *flow*.

Flow is what the groundbreaking Hungarian psychologist Mihaly Csikszentmihalyi explains as "the state in which people are so involved in an activity that nothing else seems to matter." The experience of said activity—swimming, say, or playing music—is so entirely enjoyable, he says, "that people will do it even at great cost, for the sheer sake of doing it." I think of frigid waters, crack-of-dawn workouts, shoulder injuries, all the money I've spent on bikinis.

Nearly three decades ago, Csikszentmihalyi was the first to use the word *flow* to describe the experience of being so totally immersed that the self seems to fall away, along with any awareness of the passage of time. "Every action, movement, and thought follows inevitably from the previous one, like playing jazz," he writes. This kind of effortless, deeply engaged concentration is joyful. For me, actually getting into water to chase that ecstatic state of mind has a double appeal: it's two kinds of immersion experienced at once.

In 1810, a century and a half before Csikszentmihalyi defined flow as such, the poet Lord Byron swam the Hellespont, the treacherous four-mile strait that is today known as the Dardanelles, in northern Turkey. He crossed from the Aegean to the Sea of Marmara, swimming with the tide from Europe to Asia. In the process, he kicked off a centuries-long fascination with the waters there. To this day, swimmers are enamored with the traverse of these symbolic seas. But what I'm most interested in is the idea that this swim is the thing that unclogged Byron's creative faucet.

Byron was obsessed with swimming. He suffered from a leg deformity, which severely contracted his gait; he never felt so free and himself as when he was in the water. "I delight in the sea," he wrote, "and come out with a buoyancy of spirits I never feel on any other occasion." He entertained the thought of having been a merman in a previous life. He swam wherever he could: bridge to bridge on the Thames River, in a Tagus River estuary in Lisbon, down the length of Venice's Grand Canal. At the time of his Hellespont swim, he had published some poetry but had not yet established himself as one of the great Romantic poets.

His successful Hellespont crossing, though, got his muse talking, and he produced "Written after Swimming from Sestos to Abydos," a satiric poem in homage to the swim and to the Greek myth of Hero and Leander. Leander, a young man from Abydos, falls in love with Hero, a priestess of Aphrodite who lives in a tower in Sestos. Every night, Leander swims the four miles of the Hellespont to visit Hero, guided by her lamp. One night the lamp blows out, and he drowns, overcome by the waves and currents. She throws herself from her tower to join him in death.

Of the strenuous swim, Byron wrote airily of the divergence in consequence for the lovers and himself:

'Twere hard to say who fared the best:
Sad mortals! thus the Gods still plague you!
He lost his labour, I my jest:
For he was drown'd, and I've the ague.

Yes, Byron escaped with a bout of fever and chills, but for all his jaunty tone, he felt that swimming coaxed him out of melancholy, opened up his creative stores, and gave him access to his best self. In truth, the Hellespont became a touchstone for him. In 1819, he would write the first two cantos of "Don Juan," his poetic masterpiece; in it, he makes more proud references to that crossing. He also wrote many imaginative letters to friends riffing on the Hero and Leander myth as it related to his swim. Eventually, Byron joined Greece's war of independence against the Ottoman Empire, for which he would become a Greek national hero.

In time, "Byronic" would be a label for our most passionate seekers, swimmers, and artists. Byron came to represent what the cultural historian Jacques Barzun once described as a "concentrated mind," as well as "high spirits, wit, daylight good sense, and a passion for truth—in short a unique discharge of intellectual vitality." Swimming the Hellespont was the thing that loosed Byron's imagination; only after did his words, and his world, generate a vivid electricity potent enough to reach the rest of us.

15

A Religious Exercise

The focused immediacy of swimming encourages a mindset that reminds me of how my young children think: it's an ever-present-ness. Every past moment is immediately replaced by a new one: a constant stream of *now*, and *now*, and *now* that doesn't allow much room to dwell too long on things past, or what's to come. Living in the now is a state of being that my busy brain finds challenging—but I desire it. Swimming is an antidote for the existential anxiety from which I suffer.

In *Waterlog*, his celebrated chronicle of swimming through Britain's waterways, the naturalist Roger Deakin described swimming as having a transformative, *Alice-in-Wonderland* quality; it was an activity that had power over his perception of self and of time. "When you enter the water, something like metamorphosis happens," he wrote. "Leaving behind the land, you go through the looking-glass surface and enter a new world . . . You see and experience things when you're swimming in a way that is completely different from any other." Your sense of the present, he added, "is overwhelming."

Athletes often talk about "being in the zone," where performance seems to happen at an automatic level. Researchers have described this as a psychological alteration of time that pulls your focus to the here and now—you're so consumed by the activity, and so occupied with reading and reacting to external stimuli, that time seems to slow down, so that the present moment is expanded.

The psychologist Robert Nideffer, who first helped establish sports psychology as a discipline in the 1980s, has defined *zone* and *flow* as two similar, but distinct, immersive states—using *zone* to refer to the optimal state of *physical* performance and *flow* to refer to the optimal state of *mental* performance. People who are in the zone, he argues, experience time as slowed down. People who are in a flow state, by contrast, lose awareness of time, so that it seems to fly by.

For the athlete, of course, attention to physical performance is all-consuming; in a race, the point is to go fast, so the brain can't wander too far from that objective. This is the type of Navy SEAL laser focus that Ledecky and Phelps excel at. Even for me, a mere mortal in the pool, competition fastens my attention so tightly to the action that it creates a kind of tunnel vision. The neuropsychologist David Eagleman has determined that this slowing-of-time perception comes from memories being formed more richly during high-adrenaline, high-stress events—whether it's a competition or a near-death experience. (Racing, after all, is the sublimation of our survival instincts into a competition.) In retrospect, we remember those events in greater detail, so that time *seems* expanded, and thereby slowed down.

Absent a race situation, or one in which water is a threat, though, I've found that the refinement of movement to automation is actually the thing that allows my attention to shift elsewhere. While competition itself is at odds with flow, the training part enables it. When you've reached fluency, that physical ease and pleasure grants your mind entry to uncharted territory. Push through the looking-glass, and you'll discover a different way of being. This heightened attentiveness—the ballooning of time, or the speeding-up of it; the perception that time no longer matters, or that it matters less than you might have thought—is the kind of flow I'm after.

As human swimmers, we can never really *be* the fish. You and I, we know that. We don't have to remind ourselves that it's water around us. But we get *glimpses* of what it's like to be the fish. We get flashes of forgetting the water. In the forgetting, we can drift. Daydreaming is critical to problem solving and creativity. Scientists now know that when our minds are wandering without any particular external focus, the brain's "default-mode network" is active. It's what makes fresh, unexpected connections possible. And it's the reason you get some of your best ideas in the shower. The marine biologist and author Wallace J. Nichols is an evangelist of achieving what he calls "blue mind," which emphasizes the importance of drifting to discovery, and water as a way to enable that process. "Being around water provides a sensory-rich environment with enough 'soft fascination' to let our focused attention rest and the default-mode network to kick in," he writes. "It's no coincidence that Archimedes was in the bathtub when he deduced a method for measuring the volume of an object with an irregular shape. *Eureka!*"

In its power to produce an altered state, Lynne Cox explains to me, swimming is like a drug. Sometimes we zero in on something with unparalleled lucidity, and we gain the ability to tune out the extraneous stuff; other times the focus is fuzzy, and one thought leads to another, without interruption. "Who needs psychedelics," she says with a laugh, "when you can just go for a swim in the ocean?"

The late neurologist and writer Oliver Sacks described a transcendent state that is accessible to all, from his father—with his "great whalelike bulk," who swam daily and elegantly until ninety-four years of age—to the very young. Sacks wrote books in his head while swimming. Cox became great friends with Sacks, and on the occasions that they ended up in New York or California at the same time, they would go for swims together. During their first meeting, they shared a lane in a Manhattan pool. Afterward, Sacks climbed out of the pool, still dripping, to write notes on a waterproof tablet.

Cox noticed. She told him that she, too, came up with her best brainstorms while swimming. They agreed that swimming was an ideal time to ruminate, to noodle for noodling's sake, to compose in one's head.

What is it like inside Cox's head when she's swimming?

"It's a state between a dream state and an awake state," she tells me. Maybe, she says, we can call it *sea-dreaming*. The rhythm of swimming lulls your body—which, well-trained, seems to keep moving on its own—and your brain is allowed to go wherever it wants.

"Maybe you smell the coffee someone is drinking on the pier," Cox says. "There's this awareness of the ripples of water, the pelicans sliding right by. Maybe your heart stops as you see a wave of silvery anchovies swimming below you." In the hushed oceanic roar, you can choose to filter some things out and to focus on others. Cognitive scientists have shown that water sounds—the rhythmic hum of the ocean, the rush of a waterfall—are calming to the human brain. We experience a drop in heart rate and blood pressure and an increase in alpha-wave activity—those brain wavelengths associated with relaxation and boosted serotonin—as well as that creative thinking. While tooling around on Spotify one day, I find that white-noise water sounds are some of the biggest hits on the music-streaming service; one such track, called "Rolling Ocean Waves," has been played nearly fifteen million times.

Walks in the woods are all well and good, as Thoreau illustrated in his transcendentalist classic, *Walden*. But during the two years, two months, and two days that he spent living in that cabin at Walden Pond, between 1845 and 1847, he also got up early every morning to swim; he described it as "a religious exercise, and one of the best things which I did." Each of his swims stimulated body and mind. Each day's routine of rousing early to do so was a way to enact his desire to "live deliberately" in the New England forest.

Much has been made of the walk as the instrument for big thinkers: Charles Darwin; Albert Einstein; Amos Tversky and Daniel Kahneman, who famously rambled together and revolutionized the science of decision making. Less has been explicitly made of swimming—a similar kind of aid, more medium than tool—for channeling the inner life and improving the flow of thoughts. (Though Einstein could not swim, he loved to journey by water. In his travel diaries, dating from 1922 to 1923 but just recently published, he wrote, "How conducive to thinking and working the sea voyage is—a paradisaical state without correspondence, visits, meetings, and other inventions of the devil!")

The physical action matters just as much as the environment does. "The way we move our bodies further changes the nature of our thoughts, and vice versa," notes the science journalist Ferris Jabr, in an essay called "Why Walking Helps Us Think." It follows that the pace of swimming, because of its fluid continuity, encourages a specific kind of thinking. There are the same changes to our body chemistry in swimming as there are in land exercise: faster heartbeat, increased circulation, more blood and oxygen to muscles and brain.

Jabr invokes the peripatetics of Clarissa Dalloway, Virginia Woolf's classic musing, ambulatory character, as someone who "does not merely perceive the city around her. Rather, she dips in and out of her past." Woolf herself, writing in her diary about the stimulating energy of walking through

London, used energetic, aquatic language to describe the immersive experience as "being on the highest crest of the biggest wave, right in the centre & swim of things."

In his detailing of Stanford University research experiments on the relationship between walking and creativity, Jabr writes that walking set "the mind adrift on a frothing sea of thought." For Jabr, Woolf, and others, the choice of words betrays them. They talk of "ideas bubbling up," the tumbling of them, the "wrinkling water" in a current of thought. Walking is conducive to thinking, but swimming is just as true a conduit.

To live deliberately as a swimmer means that you are a seeker: a chaser of the ocean's blue corduroy, a follower of river veins. The science writer Florence Williams notes that "place matters"—something that poets and philosophers from Aristotle to Wordsworth have been telling us for ages. "Our nervous systems are built to resonate with set points in the environment," Williams writes, in her book *The Nature Fix*. "Science is now bearing out what the Romantics knew to be true." Byron knew it, and swam after it whenever he could. We want to be near the ocean, the lake, the river. We build houses on the beach despite hurricane warnings and sea-level rise because that view does something to us.

Hospital patients recovering from heart surgery have been found to need less pain medication when there are nature scenes at the foot of their beds; an image that includes water is even more effective than an image of an enclosed forest in reducing anxiety during the post-operative period. As humans, we need doses of nature, and because "our brains especially love water," Williams writes, we need more "blue space," not just green space, in our urban areas. Williams gives a shout-out to the aquatic specialness of the San Francisco Bay Area—all those South End and Dolphin Club swimmers, stroking to Alcatraz!—but reserves her greatest admiration for Wellington, New Zealand, which has a *public snorkel trail*. (Book your tickets now.)

During one of their swims, Cox asked Sacks if she could give him a tip or two on his backstroke. He was happy and agreeable about it, because anything that allowed him to swim more easily meant that he could swim without having to devote too much mental bandwidth to the act, freeing his mind to puzzle over other things.

In 2015, Sacks was eighty-two and dying of cancer. And yet he still swam a mile a day, for as long as he could, writing until the end.

JOY IS, QUITE simply, essential to the achievement of the flow state. Both Nideffer and Csikszentmihalyi emphasize that the psychological challenge has to be something we love doing, or we can't get there.

As much as I try to stick with scientists and studies in the examination of flow, I can't help but turn back to the poets for the most convincing evidence of swimming's perks. Swimming can lead to creative output and discovery, certainly, but it is also a way to change your mood, because when you get down to it, flow is nothing if it's not getting lost in the sensory pleasure of the thing.

A rural New Hampshire farm was home to Maxine Kumin, a Pulitzer Prize–winning poet who died in 2014. She was also a swimmer—lucky for us. Her particular swimming history included stints as an instructor at a summer camp and captain of the swim team at Radcliffe College. In an early poem titled "Junior Life Saving," she summoned up the wild angles and textures of kids by a lake in summer, from the "isosceles of knees" to their "sun-killed skin." The lake itself is sentient, witty; it has timing. It "smiles to a fish / and quiets back to glass." Swimming, to the children, is magic; she hates to tell them of the perils of that water, hates to watch the magic seep away. But she does it still; it's her job. She teaches them the skills they need to keep themselves, and that magic, alive.

Later in life, Kumin wrote of solitary daily swims in what she called her "invented puddle," a pond she and her husband had dug into the marshland of their New Hampshire property in 1963. She loved that pond and swam in it as much as she could. She watched it freeze in winter, the ice cracking "like target practice"; in spring, she watched the tadpoles "quake from the jello / and come into being." The otter, she observed, is a spectacular swimmer. She likened the "cupping and pull / of handholds on water" to the rhythm of a song. The soundtrack of a swim: it was an idea she kept returning to, again and again, in different works, over the decades.

Kumin's most famous and iconic poem, "Morning Swim," was also her favorite:

> Fish twitched beneath me, quick and tame
> In their green zone they sang my name
>
> and in the rhythm of the swim
> I hummed a two-four-time slow hymn.

Here, she writes of the musicality of that swim. The fish have a beat, and so does she as she kicks her feet. The beauty comes from the rightness of timing, everything in sync, from breath to bubbles. In this falling into synchronicity between the body and the environment, the dividing line between the two ceases to exist. Swimming is something that requires us to make our bodies a part of another body unlike ours, that of water. She notes that as she enters the water, the water enters her. The conjoining is complete.

Reading Kumin helps me realize how much swimming is an unflinching giving-over to an element. Her record of the pleasures amplifies my own awareness of what absorbs me when I swim. Something as simple as rounding a rocky promontory into a breath-stealing change in temperature. *What does it feel like?* Something as simple as looking at brook trout, the mister followed by the missus. *Where are they going?* Something as simple as diving in from rocks and aiming to come up "into the fizz / of lime-green light." *Will I emerge transformed?*

In these small moments of observation, there is frozen time. In the period that I'm writing this, I visit a woodsy old resort area in Sonoma County with two friends and go swimming in the Russian River. It's late spring and dry in Northern California, the midday sun hot, the mosquitoes already whining, but the breeze ruffles the tree canopy and hints at the cool evening to come. Entry into that slash of green water is brisk but not unwelcome—more like a friendly pat on the bottom, a little wake-up, than a rude punch to the face. I swim round the pebbled bend and turn upstream. Suddenly it's as if I'm swimming on a treadmill—one of those Endless Pools with the constant current that holds you in place. I notice the leaves zipping by even as I swim, carried past me by the rushing water. I keep stroking, looking down, and see little twigs flying by. If I stop swimming, the incremental forward progress instantly becomes backward progress, and the upstream bend in the river recedes with shocking speed.

I experiment with the hydro-economy of my movements: swimming to hold position, pausing to drift back downstream. Swim to hold, pause to drift. Finally, I stop swimming altogether, holding my arms in front of me as I soar above the rippled river bottom. A fish flicks its tail into the depths, and then I turn onto my back to watch the sky rip by. I am alone, but I don't feel lonely. Out here in the river, to swim is to be a part of things.

16

The Liquid State

What do we think about when we're swimming? Unlike land-based exercise, swimming requires submersion and that characteristic isolation. But isolation in this context is a rare blessing. In the always-connected modern age, the medium represents a means of disappearing. Each pool is in fact a potential portal.

Sometimes swimming is a wormhole through which to escape the grinding machinery of everyday life. I get in a lake and swim away, as far as I can. When I get far enough away, literally and figuratively, I know it, because I find I want to go back. It's an exercise in thresholds. How much I can take, how much distance I need, how far I can get from shore before I feel afraid, at what point I desire to return to land. I brew and brood over things that seem to be of consequence, but by the end of a swim, the water has washed much of that away. I come out with my mood and mental clarity improved by a minimum of 48 percent.

Cold metallic sky on a fall morning, cool rain dimpling the surface of the pool. I cruise along in backstroke, feeling the here-and-nowness of the warm water. A crow flies across my field of vision. *How many birds poop in the pool each day?* This is not the most profound thought I've ever had while swimming, but it's a favorite nonetheless. Birds fly overhead all the time. They poop quite frequently. We see the evidence of this on our driveways, on our cars, in the school parking lot. *What about when they let fly over a body of water? What about over my body, in water? When, and how often, does this happen?* I follow the skip and jump of my mind to the edge of the pool and into the gutter, where I hope the poop ends up. I find that I'm delighted to be ruminating on bird shit. The pleasure of this whole processional of thought stems from its curious novelty: the unexpected left turns, the thinking for thinking's sake. Other days, I sing songs or make to-do lists or fantasize about what I'm going to eat for breakfast. Suffice it to say that it's not just profound thought that can clear one's mind.

Most days, if I'm not in the ocean for a surf at first light, I get into the neighborhood pool by eight-thirty a.m. Even when there's frost on the ground, the water is warm. Unless you're the lifeguard, blowing the whistle when you want me to get out, I don't know you exist. For sixty blessed minutes and three thousand two hundred yards, I'm my only audience. In a pool there's nothing much to look at once the goggles fog over. I have spit and sprayed all manner of antifog fixes into them, and none has kept the mist from creeping up on my vision like cataracts. But I'm OK with that. Sound? The sloshing of water pretty much cancels out everything else. Taste and smell are largely of the chlorine and salt variety—though, at my old pool, I used to smell burgers cooking from the café downstairs. Nowadays I get whiffs of eggs and hash browns from the high-school cafeteria next door. Despite all the tech advances of the last few years, you won't see many swimmers wearing earphones or bone-conduction music devices: they just don't work that well.

Submersion creates internal quiet, too. Sometimes swimming to blankness is the goal. We enter the meditative state induced by counting laps and observe the subtle play of light as the sun moves across the lanes. We slip from thought to thought, and then there's a momentary nothingness. In that brief interlude, we are entirely liberated from the weight of thinking. When he was a child, Michael Phelps was diagnosed with ADHD; back then, the pool was his "safe haven," in part, he says, because "being in the pool slowed down my mind." More recently, in retirement, away from the stress of competition, he has talked about the pool as a place of sanctuary and renewed mental health.

In John Cheever's 1964 short story "The Swimmer," Neddy Merrill swims home through the backyard pools of his suburban neighbors. To get there, he must navigate the parties and social merriment surrounding every body of water. At one stop, Neddy "stood by the bar for a moment, anxious not to get stuck in any conversation that would delay his voyage. When he seemed about to be surrounded he dove in and swam." Water, then, is a bubble in which all social pressure is easily eluded.

Coach Jay tells me that a long swim leaves his mind calm, collected, and organized in a way that other sports don't.

"It's hard to leave the pool angry about something," he says. "It doesn't lend itself to that." As the world, with its escalating rings and pings, gets ever more hysterical, suspending yourself in water becomes ever more appealing.

"Theories and stories would construct themselves in my mind as I swam to and fro, or round and round Lake Jeff," Oliver Sacks wrote in "Water Babies," one of my favorite essays of all time. Five hundred lengths in a pool were never boring or monotonous; instead, Sacks said, "Swimming gave me a sort of joy, a sense of well-being so extreme that it became at times a sort of ecstasy." The body is engaged in full physical movement, but the mind itself floats, untethered. Beyond this, he added, "there is all the symbolism of swimming—its imaginative resonances, its mythic potentials." Echoes of Byron.

One recent weekday morning at the pool, I watch an eight-year-old boy and his teenage sister swim their laps beside me. The boy shivers on land, lips blue and knees knocking. But when he hits the water, he is confident, focused, as fluent in the medium as a seal. For a little while, there is just a boy in his buoyancy.

This is not to say that swimmers find it easy to be Zen masters. Bill Clinton once told PBS that he and Hillary swim together every afternoon; if either dares to mention a political topic during the course of their swim, he said, "We will stop the other one."

I ask Dara Torres, who has amassed countless training hours for her five Olympics, what she thinks about when she's swimming. "I'm always doing five things at once," she tells me by phone (at the time, she was driving a car). "So when I get in the water, I think about all the things that I have to do. But sometimes I go into a state—I don't really think about anything." The important thing, she says, is that the time is yours. "You can use it for anything. It depends where your head is at—it's a reflection of where you are."

The reflection of where you are: in essence, a status update to you, and only you. And the experience is egalitarian. You don't have to be a great swimmer to appreciate the benefits of sensory solitude and the equilibrium the water can bring.

Notable waters in literature, art, and movies where our imaginations have gone swimming:

The depths of the Ionian Sea, into which an angry Poseidon plunged Odysseus, who was eventually guided by the goddess Athena to a safe landing on a riverbank on Scheria, supposedly today's Corfu (Homer, *The Odyssey*, eighth century BC).

The Atlantic coast of Africa, where local water spirits blended with European iconography to produce Mami Wata, or "mother water," a mermaid deity with a double tail who swam with the African diaspora to such places as Haiti, Brazil, and the Dominican Republic (late fifteenth century).

The Tiber River, in which Cassius and Caesar once had a swimming race, and Cassius rescued a tiring Caesar, later citing it as an example of his own superiority to Caesar (William Shakespeare, *Julius Caesar*, 1599).

The Louisiana coast of the Gulf of Mexico, where Edna Pontellier teaches herself how to swim, and ultimately drowns herself, to free herself from the grim fetters of societal expectations (Kate Chopin, *The Awakening*, 1899).

A tour of the Gulf Stream, off the coast of Cuba, a three-day journey experienced by the aging fisherman Santiago while being pulled by a giant marlin who won't stop swimming (Ernest Hemingway, *The Old Man and the Sea*, 1952).

Across the Yangtze River, an actual swim by Mao Zedong that straddles fact and fiction when presented as Communist propaganda, in a poem supposedly written by the Chairman himself (Mao Zedong, "Swimming," 1956).

A backyard swimming pool in California, signifying the open canvas that is an aimless young man's life, no thought of what's next until Mrs. Robinson shows up (Mike Nichols, *The Graduate*, 1967).

A pool in the south of France, which sets the stage for the unraveling of the painter's relationship with his partner, even more meaningful when juxtaposed against that painter's iconic poolside scene of blissful gay domesticity (David Hockney, *Portrait of an Artist [Pool with Two Figures]*, 1972).

A beach in Miami as a storm rolls in, where a boy nicknamed "Little" floats in the arms of a drug dealer named Juan who is teaching him to swim, all of it making for a stirring, revelatory moment of metamorphosis (Barry Jenkins, *Moonlight*, 2016).

PEOPLE OFTEN TELL me about their swimming habits—for example, how, when they visit or move to a new city, the first thing they do is account for all the pools and open water. It's a way to get to know a place. It's how they map out unfamiliar geographies and make them their own.

When I was growing up, my father told me about Hainan Island, the "Chinese Hawaii," perched on the South China Sea. To the Chinese, Hainan has always had a romantic, frontier air about it. As the southernmost point in China, it is the only tropical island, and it served for centuries as a place of exile for poets and politicos. To my father, a Hong Kong–born painter who divorced my mother and left New York to go back and live in China, it was a dream of a place, a palm-fringed paradise that represented the ideal inspiration for him.

There was a time in my early thirties when I hadn't seen my father in three years. One morning I took a deep breath and called him up. My work would take me to Hainan that year. "Come swimming again," I said, my stomach full of butterflies. "Come meet me in the South China Sea." And he did.

The island was in the midst of a development boom, but still we were able to walk on stretches of empty white beach, with spearmint waves lapping the shores, and take drives to the rural inner parts of the island. A Chinese acquaintance back home wrote out a traditional poem for me from memory, a long verse with many characters about Hainan's famously striking landscape. "Hainan is very beautiful," he'd said. "I've never been there, but I learned about it in school." I brought the poem with me, which my friend had written in Chinese, and asked my father to translate it for me when we were in Hainan. The island's legendary mist-clad cliffs and coastlines, straight out of the old calligraphy scrolls and paintings, came to life.

I tried to forget that as a child, my father was a daily constant in my life. Once, when I was twelve, he told me I was his best friend. It hurt to remember that; as an adult, I saw him only every year or two. The first time I insisted on visiting him in China—on my way back from that college semester abroad in Australia—I screamed and cried at him, not for leaving my mother but for the way he did it. There was no swimming on that trip, but there was a pool's worth of tears.

On Hainan Island, we came together in a truce. The trip was a pilgrimage for me, to a new, more forgiving place. I coaxed him into accompanying me on a swim. He, the former lifeguard, could not remember the last time he went swimming. His butterfly wasn't half bad. The air was humid. The water was warm, enveloping, a balm. He looked happy. As I floated on my back and stared at that cloud-streaked sky over the South China Sea, I felt that I was, too.

Franz Kafka observed that "the truth is always an abyss. One must—as in a swimming pool—dare to dive from the quivering springboard of trivial everyday experience and sink into the depths, in order later to rise again—laughing and fighting for breath—to the now doubly illuminated surface of things." We dare to jump so we can see something new. And sometimes we do it to recover a sense of what we once had.

17

From One Swimmer to Another

O nce upon a time, I fell in love with a family and a lake. In the ritual of swimming, the connection of one body to another, of one *person* to another, there is flow of a different sort to be found.

The first summer we were together as a couple, Matt took me to visit his grandparents at their cottage on the northern shores of Lake George, five hours north of New York City. Ted and Shirley met on a swimming raft on that lake, in 1939, and got married after the war. Their safe harbor was the tiny hamlet of Silver Bay and the grand old YMCA resort that had been there since 1899. Matt and I were young ourselves on that visit, just out of college, and would not be married for another eight years. But that liquid-mercury lake—framed by evergreens in the picture-postcard view from the screened-in back porch—would be a touchstone from the first.

Everyone in the family had a particular way of crossing the lake. Grandpa Ted had a special affection for tooling around in fishing boats. He owned three in his life: *The Ultimate*

Folly I, II, and *III,* each larger and more elaborate than the last. No one could remember him having ever actually caught a fish.

Uncle Chris, all six feet five of him, folded himself into a kayak before paddling across. Matt's mom, Robin, loved to float around in a rubber dinghy—she wasn't a frequent lake crosser, but she was a spirited shore dabbler. Her husband, Jan, a marine surveyor, traversed the waters on a windsurfer and, later, on a stand-up paddleboard. Uncle George, a National Outdoor Leadership School instructor and all-around out-doorsman, liked to sail; Matt's little brother, Jesse, had just earned a license to pilot the thirteen-foot Boston Whaler.

One morning over breakfast and his daily crossword puzzle, Grandpa Ted casually mentioned that he and his friends used to swim the mile from Silver Bay across the lake to Diver's Rock, for generations the spot where children have made a heart-stopping jump into the water. "That was the thing to do back then, like swimming the English Channel," he said, his eyes sliding over to me before returning to the crossword, each completed square lettered in unwavering ink. "If you said you'd swum across the lake that day, that was something."

My ears perked up. I smiled back at him. This was something I knew how to do, and he knew it. I loved the idea of joining the generations of lake crossers before me, in a way that was *me.* He was handing me a personal invitation.

That afternoon, we pushed off from Silver Bay, Matt

swimming and me beside him, paddling Grandma Shirley's old blue kayak, so he wouldn't get run over by speedboats.

We made our way out past the sailboats and motorboats bobbing in the harbor; past the raft at Bay Beach, where Ted and Shirley first set eyes on each other; past the tiny island of Scotch Bonnet, where Matt's parents were married; past a man in a boat who yelled at us through a megaphone, "Swimming in the lake is hazardous to your health," what with all the boats and Jet Skis racing about. Forty-five minutes later, we arrived at Diver's Rock, the stone-faced cliff where each member of Matt's family has made the jump. It was a veritable water tour of his family history at Lake George.

After we performed the solemn ceremony of jumping off the ledge, it was my turn to swim back across the lake. I tried not to think of speedboats and trusted my man in the blue kayak to keep me safe. The water was pancake-flat and perfect. When I beached myself on the shores of Silver Bay, I felt initiated. I thought I finally understood something about what the place meant to Matt and to the company of lake crossers before us.

Eight years later, we continued our Lake George swim, the day after our wedding, with forty of our closest friends in the flotilla. Both sets of our maternal grandparents were there to witness it, and I suppose you could say that I swam from one family into another. We returned, year after year. Even after we moved across the country to San Francisco, we kept going back—sometimes in fall or winter, mostly in summer. There have been variations on the swim. One New Year's Day, our bare feet stinging in the snow, Matt and I held the first and only meeting of the Silver Bay Polar Bear Swim Club (total members: two).

In the years since, Grandpa has gone. Jesse, too. When we go back now, it's the fireflies and the stars that get me every time. Much of modern life is filtered out through the dense trees and mountains on the winding approach to the lake. Those winking lights, bobbing along the ground and filling up the night sky with their impossible density, send a signal. It's a reminder to slow up and be awake to the real connections we have while we have them.

I started out thinking that the pleasures of swimming were all about immediacy—about being in the present—but I have found that the act of swimming can serve as ritual, too. It's not just this family, and it's not just this lake. Bodies of water are shared spaces, and this is the mythology to go with it. What is Guðlaugssund, anyway, but remembrance? Why do people do it other than to feel a kinship with Guðlaugur and their fellow Icelanders? In pursuit of a great survival tale, what did I find? A swimmer-by-swimmer connection to the man himself.

When you are tuned in to the world and its forces, revelations follow. Swim with the current, and you'll feel invincible. Swim against it, and you suddenly become aware of the invisible forces against you. I want my own children to be unafraid, because they know that the current is there, because they know what to do when they face it. These are the swimming stories I carry with me.

Pablo Neruda wrote *Twenty Love Poems and a Song of Despair*, published when he was just nineteen; he uses aquatic imagery to depict the intoxicating gorgeousness of being in love, the loss of control when we're immersed in it. The ninth poem in the collection, "Drunk with Pines," is my favorite, for its vivid conjuring of a pair of swimmers caught together in the outer waves: two passionate, parallel bodies, one yielding to the other, "like a fish infinitely fastened to my soul."

What are these if not stories of love?

WHEN IT COMES to swimming, we can understand flow to mean not just the expansive, timeless state of being that Csikszentmihalyi defined but also the flood of thoughts that swimming enables, and the connection we have to each other and to the planet we inhabit.

Flow: from Old English *flówan*; from the same root *flo-* are Old Norse *flóa*, to flood, and Dutch *vloeijen*, to flow. The word holds other secrets, too. Latin *plōrāre*, to weep; Sanskrit *plu*, to swim, bathe; Old High German *flewen*, to rinse; Greek πλωειν, to swim, float. I follow the downstream movement of language, and it offers up a raft of connections: flood, weep, swim, bathe, rinse, float. Trace this lineage and it reveals an unfettering, an unburdening, whether physical—a release of the body to water, freed from its customary weight and gravity—or emotional, through a good cry, the cleansing release of tears. In the sea, a tidal flood of water traveling from thousands of miles away can absorb the small individual burst of a dam. Elation may be essential to the flow state, but so, too, is a slice of sorrow, embedded in the very history of the word itself.

Even in grief—the breakup of my parents, a miscarriage, the death of a friend—I have marked time by water. I won't linger on these sorrows, because I don't mean to say that swimming cured me of them, but I will say that swimming, in all of its permutations—in a pool, in a lake, paddling a surfboard out to sea—has always helped me come out on the other side of a difficult time. The tides keep changing, twice a day. Water is in a forever state of flux. To swim is to witness metamorphosis, in our environment, in ourselves. To swim is to accept all the myriad conditions of life.

I think back to the beginning. We float in the womb. When we first learn to swim, we first learn to float. I watch the waves roll in and how they lift us all, together. If I am floating here in San Francisco and you are floating across the Pacific in Tokyo, are we not floating together?

Thousands of miles from where Tony Cundy lives in Tokyo, his parents have a house on the southwest coast of England, where they look out over the English Channel. Whenever he's swimming in a lake or river in Japan, practicing the strokes of *Nihon eiho*, he feels that he is connected to them. The pleasure of swimming for him is in large part the space it creates to think about where he is. "However you draw the line," he tells me, "water connects you."

FOR THE PAST several years I have watched my two sons, Felix and Teddy, now eight and six, become swimmers. From the beginning, I expected fear, but I was eager and hopeful for the moment when it would give way to something else. It turned out that fear for them was fleeting, though it would register every now and then with a shift in reference point— pool to ocean, say, or warm water to cold. What came, in quick succession, was curiosity and tentative exploration; giddiness at gliding independently from the wall; leaps into the pool; spontaneous underwater somersaults. Joy.

I remember floating in the glassy ultramarine Pacific at Tunnels Beach, on the north shore of Kauai, while pregnant with Felix, my sun-warmed belly poking above the waves as I took in the rippling red-and-green cliffs of the Nā Pali Coast. Six years later, Matt and I began a sabbatical summer—a three-month break from the daily grind—back on the island, in the little north shore town of Haena. I wanted Felix to feel that buoying for himself, outside of me, fully aware of the pulse of water on his lanky young body. I wanted a kind of time travel: to hold him simultaneously in this place as a baby and a boy.

Little by little, Felix got comfortable in the gently rolling surf. He bobbed. He practiced his freestyle and his back-stroke. He looked for brilliant pink-and-blue parrotfish. Alongside the locals, he learned to bodysurf to the sand. Felix learned to love the feeling that the water there was in some way *alive* and different from the stillness of a pool. One day he befriended a stout, sun-bronzed middle-aged body-surfer named Dave who shouted encouragement and expertly propelled himself toward shore with élan and grace. That evening, my son drew a picture of himself bodysurfing in the waves with his "new friend" Dave. Years later, Felix talks about him still.

Every morning at Tunnels I swam a mile or more, zig-zagging between reefs and following the locals to what they could show me. Once I tailed two spearfishermen, clad in their dusky-green camouflage wetsuits, and spotted four large sea turtles resting at the bottom of the ocean. They were being feasted on by tiny fish known as cleaner wrasse; in a marvel of symbiosis, the wrasse detail the turtles' hard shells by hoovering up parasites and dead skin. An efficient forty-five minutes later, the young fishermen emerged from the sea with the day's catch in hand: huge mahi-mahi, two each. On other days I swam alongside ropy-armed surfers as far as I could before they paddled beyond the outer reef, where the wind whipped whitecaps across the sea. I treaded water and watched safely from within the reef as they made elegant, sinuous turns across the face of each wave as it broke.

We became friendly with a young family living nearby whom we saw often during these mornings. The toddler daughter liked to investigate our snacks and toys and played with Teddy. The father, nut-brown from the sun, sat by the sea gathering tiny, intricately patterned shells the size of baby teeth that he said were once collected only by the holiest of Hawaiian priests.

One morning as I swam in the coral-punctuated shallows, two men called my attention to a four-foot shark resting on its side in the waist-deep water. It was a juvenile, they said, and it had probably died while trying to find its way back to deeper water through the maze of vividly colored near-shore corals—some boulder-size, others cactuslike, still others resembling giant brains with lobes.

Later, a lifeguard in sunglasses and red swim trunks roared up in a dune buggy and dragged the shark up onto the beach. Bystanders came around to stare at its smooth gray hide, bloodied nose, and clouded-over eyes. The episode didn't stop any of us from swimming, but it was yet another sobering reminder, welcome or not, of the ocean's ever-present dangers: sharks, riptides, razor-sharp reefs.

As an adult, I have come to appreciate water—an ocean, a lake, a pool—as a mode of inner as well as outer transport. In the middle of Honolulu, one of my favorite swimming spots is Ala Moana Beach, along the downtown waterfront. In the middle of the city, steps from high-rise towers, the glassy, reef-protected ocean at Ala Moana serves as the de facto communal pool. To swim there is to experience the place at water level: Turn your head *makai*, toward the ocean, to breathe, and there are surfers paddling out to the break; turn your head *mauka*, toward the mountains, and there are Japanese brides and grooms having pictures taken on their wedding day. From this perspective, everything feels strangely possible.

WHY DO I swim? Many pages ago, I said that I was a character in this book, too. But maybe it's the opposite: swimming has always played a central role in my life—constant but mercurial, a shape-shifter.

I have written about survival, well-being, community, competition, and flow as separate streams of reasoning. But in truth, they all run together. A swim can take different forms, different moods, and different functions, depending on the time of day, the time of year, the time of life. It can cast light, or filter it, or block it altogether. It can be energizing or enervating. It can pull me to a place of comfort or push me to a place of fear. It can remind me, through ritual, or help me forget, through flow.

Swimming helps me to slow down, and to speed up. I have practiced enough to know how to be calm, and how to generate controlled fury. I can forget myself in a bathtub-warm lake or, in a steam-wisped Icelandic lagoon, be so exquisitely present that every glint and glimmer is seared into my brain forever.

Here is the writer Rebecca Solnit on the color blue: it is, bewitchingly, "the color of there seen from here, the color of where you are not." There is a seductiveness to water. From afar, it gleams and glistens, a shiny liquid jewel. It is inviting. It swirls, fans, and coalesces, embracing you. It holds you and yet cannot be held by you. When we immerse ourselves, something is awakened. It is as if eyesight has been turned on, or hearing. It is a vital new sense discovered. When I was a teenage lifeguard, I once saved a little girl from drowning. Those eyes, underwater, big as dinner plates. As I towed her to the side of the diving tank, the tensed muscles of her body made her feel remarkably heavy for such a small, skinny child. She got out of the pool and promptly burst into tears. When her brothers and sisters ran over, they exclaimed that she didn't know how to swim. "Why did you jump in if you don't know how to swim?" I asked her, gently. Her only answer was more tears.

As the girl's siblings bundled her away in a towel and comforted her, an old awareness surfaced in me, recalling myself on that long-ago day at Jones Beach. Drowning is quiet and quick. Someone might notice—or no one might. It strikes me now that we responders are moved to ask, *Why? Why jump in if you can't swim? Why endanger yourself so illogically?* The little girl couldn't explain it, just as I couldn't put into words what I felt when I was her age, tumbling in the surf. But I know the answer now.

Blue: the color of where you are not.

Wherever it is I might be in my head, the winking where-you-are-not-ness of water issues an invitation to go elsewhere. It's an escape from Earth's terra firma, with regularly scheduled departures. I am reminded of it every time I slip into an unfamiliar body of water, eager to see the way it behaves once I enter its liquid mass. Will it absorb me easily, imperturbably, or will it chop, splash, resist with every stroke? The soft, muted salt of a pool is different from the gritty mineral flavor of the sea. So is the mint-candy look of the Caribbean versus the cobalt vastness of the Aegean. I want to try all the flavors; I think my thirst for them is what Neruda called "my solid marine madness."

This color-saturated expansion of life goes beyond the natural world to encompass the man-made. On a flight to Palm Springs, I see the geometry of pool-centric living clearly laid out below in the repeating grid of turquoise rectangles, ovals, and odd little squiggles. Pools can be anywhere and are especially necessary in a land-locked locale. Enter and you may go anywhere in your thoughts; enter in the specific geography of Southern California, for example, and you gain insight into the American optimism of the post–World War II era. This is where Hollywood once went to get away, where people found escape by diving in; the very idea of these sapphire pools as escape infiltrated the iconography of American film and literature. Or take a dip in a hot pool in Iceland in the dead of winter, and you'll see through a crack, the delicious warmth reviving you to the nocturnal pleasures of the once-forbidding dark. We have put pools in places where they are necessary for surviving the pressures of modern life. Pools are a symbol. It is possible to emerge from the water reinvented, a new version of yourself.

In a typical pool, the distance between the diving board and the ladder is twenty feet, maybe, but so much more separates the two. In that space, we might catch a glimpse of what we desire. I remember the summer Felix jumped off a diving board for the first time. As he stood there on the plank gathering courage, I saw an ocean of possibility open up in the space that separated his tiny, dripping body from the water below. He sprang toward the ladder at the side of the diving tank, and I saw myself reflected in the water, in him, as he took flight, arms outstretched, suspended there for one glorious moment. What did I wish for him? An elemental understanding of water, of how it can be a portal to somewhere else. He hit the water with a muted, backlit splash. When he bobbed up to the surface, he paused, just for a heartbeat. Then he began to swim.

EPILOGUE

~

In early May 2018, Kim Chambers was diagnosed with Guillain-Barré syndrome, a rare neurological disorder in which the body's immune system attacks the nerves, causing numbness and paralysis that can quickly spread across the entire body. The paralysis started one morning in Kim's left foot, but it crept up to her legs and arms so rapidly that when she finally consented to go to the emergency room, she was struggling for breath. Later, the doctors told Kim that she had been ninety minutes away from respiratory paralysis—had she not gone to the hospital when she did, she would have suffocated. When she left the intensive-care ward, she was paralyzed from the waist down and had trouble speaking. The cause of Guillain-Barré is unknown, and there is no cure; about 80 percent of adults recovering from the illness can walk independently six months after diagnosis, and about 60 percent fully recover motor strength in a year.

Five weeks after Kim entered the hospital, she was back in San Francisco Bay on the occasion of her forty-first birthday: a five-minute immersion that required one wheelchair, a three-hour recovery nap, and an endless circle of friends. The body, she says, follows the mind. For the second time in her life, she has thrown herself into full-time physical therapy to relearn how to walk again. Fatigue, lingering paralysis, and nerve pain, though, are reminders to take a moment to look up every now and again. "With my first medical mis-adventure, I became a swimmer," she tells me. "It was the best thing that happened to me. So with this latest one, I just know there's something else amazing down the line. And I'm humbled to find out what it is." She says that the moment where you begin, when you commit to yourself, is the scariest moment: jumping into the pool for the first time after almost losing a leg, or jumping off a boat at the Farallon Islands on a dense, ink-black night, unsure if the landing zone is right in the mouth of a great white shark. But Kim is jumping into this new life with both eyes open. And, as with the first time around, she has found the water to be a willing midwife to her rebirth.

ACKNOWLEDGMENTS

This book came into being with the kindness and longtime support of many extraordinary people. My greatest thanks to those who so generously shared their time and their swimming lives with me—in particular Guðlaugur Friðþórsson, who invited me into his home with an open heart; Kim Chambers, who told me her story with such infectious joy and wonder; Jay Taylor, who remains my most faithful pen pal; and Midori Ishibiki, who introduced me to the miraculous world of samurai swimming.

Over the course of reporting I asked a lot of busy people a lot of annoying questions, and they entertained my queries with nothing but patient consideration. Special thanks to the scientists—Paul Sereno, Hirofumi Tanaka, Shingo Kajimura, Chris Stringer, Renato Bender, Nicole Bender, Melanie Rudd, Anna Gislén—and to filmmaker Elena Kubarska, who helped me paint a picture of the Bajau depicted in her documentary *Walking Under Water*. I got to bug my swimming heroes about what they think about when they're swimming: Dara Torres, Lynne Cox, Lewis Pugh, Ram Barkai. Thank you to Bruce Gemmell and Jim Bauman for opening a window into the athlete's brain. Huge thanks also to the indefatigable Alan Allison for his help with the Guðlaugssund archives and to Helga Hallbergsdóttir of the Vestmannaeyjar History Museum.

Thank you to Aaron Retica, for suggesting I write the essay that started it all. Thanks to my early readers: Sara Houghteling, James Wilson, Ethan Watters, Andrea Walker, Caroline Paul. You cheered me on, offered advice at critical junctures, and kept me believing. To Civil Twilight—Caroline, Sarah McCarthy, and Harper Honan—I thank you for all the dawn patrols. You keep me happy, sane, and taking the high line, in surfing and in life.

To Rachel Levin, my work wife, hotel wife, sister: I'm forever grateful for our long walks and your bighearted friendship. Your smart, spirited feedback buoys me every step of the way. To Chris Colin, my work husband and co-writing buddy . . . thank you for bringing your humor, music, and clear-eyed thoughtfulness to the table. I am sharper for it.

My deepest gratitude to Danielle Svetcov, incredible agent, elemental force, all-around wonderful human. I am giddy every day to know you're in my corner.

So many of the aforementioned folks came into my life because of the San Francisco Writers' Grotto, the best writing community a girl could hope for. The Grotto has been and continues to be a port in the storm of life. Special thanks to swimmers and writing neighbors Todd Oppenheimer, Bridget Quinn, Joshua Mohr, and Matthew Zapruder.

Thanks to Rebecca Skloot for bringing me into the Notto fold, where good conversation, the essential fuel to any creative endeavor, is always on tap (I'm talking to you, bright spots: Laurel Braitman, Mary Roach, Malia Wollan).

A waterfall of thanks to Amy Gash, my marvelous editor: I'm so lucky to have you. Your smarts and sharp eyes helped shape this book into the best it could be. I am over the moon to be part of the Algonquin family; you all saw my vision and believed in it from the start. So many swimmers among you! Craig Popelars, we are kin (moving to Portland only makes you closer). Thank you to Brunson Hoole, for making the train run on time, and to Kelly Policelli, for working your copy magic. Huge thanks to Jason Heuer, who made the most gorgeous book jacket, and to Steve Godwin, who designed the elegant pages within. Thank you to Michael McKenzie and Stephanie Mendoza for helping to introduce this book to the world.

All would not be complete without heartfelt shout-outs to dear friends: Tom Davidson, my earliest writing buddy and in-house neuroscience consultant; Steve Dawson, cheerful enthusiast in all things open water; Jenny Fu, Lynsay Skiba, Melissa Gibson, Esther Chak, Anna Vella, Mara Gladstone, Michele Boruta, for lifting me when I felt most heavy.

Many people told me stories that didn't make it into the book; I wish I could include them all. Helen Garcia, Kathe Rothacher, Jane Coulter, Barbara Stark Jordan, Nancy Brown . . . and Krystel Poyeton, the mayor of my pool! Merci beaucoup. It takes time for ideas to percolate, and I thank my editors, particularly at the *New York Times*, for providing me with generous opportunities to work those thoughts out in different forms over the years.

Warm gratitude to Linda and Bob Balzan, for sharing your Bolinas cottage: it inspires our family always.

To my coaches, then (Coaches Nancy, Rob, Kevin, Kathleen!) and now (Coaches Carol, Keith, and Lessly, I swear I'm coming to practice once this dang book is out).

To Andy, Stephen, Chris: you're my forever team.

To my parents, who taught me to love water.

And dearest love and thanks to my three most important boys. Felix and Teddy, you bring joy to my life every day, in the water and out of it. And to my husband, Matt, bless you for saying yes to swimming across Lake George with me, just because Grandpa said we could. There's no one I'd rather have in my polar bear club of two. I love you.

NOTES

~

SURVIVAL

1. Stone Age Swimming

3 *Late on the evening of March 11, 1984*   I spoke with Guðlaugur Friðþórsson personally about his experiences, and his story was widely reported in Icelandic and English-language newspapers and other media. "The Light in the Islands Were His Guiding Light," *Morgunblaðið*, March 12, 2004.

4 *less than a half an hour before hypothermia claimed them*   Coco Ballantyne, "Hypothermia: How Long Can Someone Survive in Frigid Water?," *Scientific American*, January 16, 2009.

5 *he showed no signs of hypothermia, only dehydration*   "Why the Fat Icelander Survived His Arctic Swim," *New Scientist*, January 23, 1986.

5 *insulated by fourteen millimeters of fat*   "Exceptional Case of Survival in Cold Water," *British Medical Journal* 292 (January 18, 1986).

6 *40 percent of the global population lives*   United Nations, "Factsheet: People and Oceans," Oceans Conference, June 2017, https://www.un.org/sustainabledevelopment/wp-content/uploads/2017/05/Ocean-fact-sheet-package.pdf.

11 *most every season, April through November*   Tara Duggan, "California Abalone Season Sunk until 2021 to Give Stressed Population Time to Rebuild," *San Francisco Chronicle*, December 13, 2018.

12 *every cove along this part of the coast* John Branch, "Prized but Perilous Catch," *New York Times*, July 27, 2014.

13 *The first known record of swimming* "Cave of Swimmers, Egypt," The British Museum, https://africanrockart .britishmuseum.org/country/egypt/cave-of-swimmers/ (accessed April 13, 2019); "Exploring the Rock Art of Gilf Kebir," Bradshaw Foundation, http://www.bradshawfoundation.com/africa/gilf_ kebir_cave_of_swimmers/index.php (accessed April 13, 2019); Stathis Avramidis, "World Art on Swimming," *International Journal of Aquatic Research and Education* 5 (2011).

14 *a time when the Sahara was green* Peter deMenocal and Jessica Tierney, "Green Sahara: African Humid Periods Paced by Earth's Orbital Changes," *Nature Education Knowledge* 3, no. 10.

14 *I read about a paleontologist named Paul Sereno* Peter Gwin, "Lost Tribes of the Green Sahara," *National Geographic*, September 2008; National Geographic Society, "Stone Age Graveyard Reveals Lifestyles of a 'Green Sahara,'" *ScienceDaily*, August 15, 2008, https://www.sciencedaily.com/releases/2008/08/ 080815101317.htm.

15 Spinosaurus aegyptiacus *as the first known swimming dinosaur* Helen Thompson, "Meet the Mighty Spinosaurus, the First Dinosaur Adapted for Swimming," *Smithsonian*, September 11, 2014.

15 *one of* People *magazine's "50 Most Beautiful People"* People, "50 Most Beautiful People of 1997," May 12, 1997.

17 *Nile perch, a freshwater monstrosity* Jennifer Blake, "Introduced Species Summary: Nile Perch (*Lates niloticus*)," Columbia University, http://www.columbia.edu/itc/cerc/danoff-burg/ invasion_bio/inv_spp_summ/Lates_niloticus.htm (accessed April 13, 2019).

20 *began to evolve nearly two hundred thousand years ago* "Human Origins," Smithsonian National Museum of Natural History, http://www.humanorigins.si.edu (accessed April 13, 2019).

20 *evidence of those ancestral humans going to sea* Andrew Lawler, "Neandertals, Stone Age People May Have Voyaged the Mediterranean," *Science*, April 24, 2018.

21 *Neanderthals, who overlapped with modern humans* Chris Stringer, "Neanderthal Exploitation of Marine Mammals in Gibraltar," *PNAS* 105 (September 22, 2008).

23 *By 2030, the number of people affected by floods* Claire Marshall, "Global Flood Toll to Triple by 2030," BBC, March 5, 2015.

24 *In California, where I live* G. Griggs et al. (California Ocean Protection Council Science Advisory Team Working Group), *Rising Seas in California: An Update on Sea-Level Rise Science*, California Ocean Science Trust, April 2017, http://www.opc .ca.gov/webmaster/ftp/pdf/docs/rising-seas-in-california-an-update-on-sea-level-rise-science.pdf; Kurtis Alexander, "Climate Change Report: California to See 77 Percent More Land Burned," *San Francisco Chronicle,* August 27, 2018.

24 *Worldwide, sea level rise has the potential* Jennifer Senior, "Not if the Seas Rise, but When and How High," *New York Times*, November 22, 2017.

2. You're a Land Animal

25 *Most land mammals possess instinctive swimming ability* Josh Gabbatiss, "The Strange Experiments That Revealed Most Mammals Can Swim," *BBC Earth*, March 21, 2017.

25 *Humans and other large primates* Renato Bender and Nicole Bender, "Swimming and Diving Behavior in Apes," *American Journal of Physical Anthropology* 152 (2013).

26 *the baby will hold her breath* E. Goksor et al., "Bradycardic Response during Submersion in Infant Swimming," *Acta Pediatrica* 91, no. 3 (March 2002); Kate Gammon, "Born to Swim?," *Popular Science*, March 6, 2014.

28 *a cork life jacket, described by Plutarch* Plutarch, "The Life of Camillus," in *The Parallel Lives*, vol. 2, Loeb Classical Library (Cambridge, MA: Harvard University Press, 1914).

28 *translucent outer layer of a tortoise shell* "The History of Goggles," The International Swimming Hall of Fame, http://www .ishof.org/assets/the-history-of-swimming-goggles.pdf (accessed April 13, 2019).

28 *a bladder constructed of animal skin* "Diving Apparatus,"
Online Gallery: Leonardo da Vinci, The British Library, http://
www.bl.uk/onlinegallery/features/leonardo/diving.html (accessed
April 13, 2019).

28 *a pulley, used by the* ama National Research Council,
Physiology of Breath-Hold Diving and the Ama of Japan: Papers
(Washington, DC: The National Academies Press, 1965), https://
doi.org/10.17226/18843.

28 *swim paddles in the shape of* Benjamin Franklin, "The Art of
Swimming," quoted in "Ben Franklin's Inventions," The Franklin
Institute, http://www.fi.edu/benjamin-franklin/inventions
(accessed April 13, 2019).

28 *a metal-framed "swimming machine"* J. Emerson, Device for
Teaching Swimming, US Patent 563,578, granted July 7, 1896,
https://patents.google.com/patent/US563578.

28 *water-wings sewn from fine cotton material* *The Publisher:
The Journal of the Publishing Industry* 89 (1908); "Deans,
'Miller Collection' rare 'Swimeesy Buoys,' original showcard
1908-1920," Vectis Auctions LTD, https://www.vectis.co.uk/
deans-inch-miller-collection-inch-rare-swimeesy-buoys-original-
showcard-1908-1920_24498 (accessed April 13, 2019).

29 *wooden swimming costume fashioned from thin strips* "New
Ideas and Inventions," *Popular Science*, May 1930; *Chop Yourself
a Piece of Bathing Suit—Wooden Swimming Outfits Make Their
Appearance at Miami—Ruth and Ruby Nolan Getting Dressed
in Their New Spruce Swimming Suits, Made of Thin Strips of
Wood* [photograph], ca. 1930, Library of Congress, Prints and
Photographs Division, Washington, DC, https://lccn.loc.gov/
96524801.

3. Lessons from a Sea Nomad

30 *swim down to two hundred feet* I spoke to Eliza Kubarska, the
director of *Walking Under Water*, a 2014 documentary about
the Bajao; Carl Zimmer, "Bodies Remodeled for a Life at Sea,"
New York Times, April 19, 2018.

31 *Moken—who also live on houseboats* Anna Gislen, "Visual
Training Improves Underwater Vision in Children," *Vision*

Research 46, no. 20 (October 2006); Brian Handwerk, "Sea Gypsies of Asia Boast 'Incredible' Underwater Vision," *National Geographic Ultimate Explorer*, May 14, 2004.

32 *the Moken survived by reading signs in the water*   "The knowledge That Saved the Sea Gypsies," *World of Science* 3, no. 2 (April-June 2005; Carrie Arnold, "Indigenous Myths Carry Warning Signals about Natural Disasters," *Aeon*, April 13, 2017.

33 *Japanese tsunami records dating back one and a half millennia* Kathryn Schulz, "The Really Big One," *New Yorker*, July 20, 2015.

34 *The last of these historically nomadic fishermen*   Human Rights Watch, *Stateless at Sea: The Moken of Burma and Thailand*, June 25, 2015, https://www.hrw.org/report/2015/06/25/stateless-sea/moken-burma-and-thailand.

34 *the naturalist Loren Eiseley wrote*   Loren Eiseley, *The Star Thrower* (New York: Harvest, 1979).

35 *all Dutch children take classes*   Michael Kimmelman, "The Dutch Have Solutions to Rising Seas. The World is Watching," *New York Times*, June 15, 2017.

4. The Human Seal

38 *Today, its fishing boats still account*   I spoke to Ragnar Arnason, a fisheries and economics professor at the University of Iceland.

38 *emblematic of the national character of Iceland*   John McPhee, "The Control of Nature: Cooling the Lava—I," *New Yorker*, February 22, 1988.

39 *Heimaey's longtime importance as a fishing port*   Statistics, events, and dates described here were largely gathered from interviews with Helga Hallbergsdóttir and from the archives at the Vestmannaeyjar History Museum.

40 *Reporters called Guðlaugur "the human seal"*   Simon Edge, "The Strange Story of the Human Seal," *Express*, July 9, 2013.

44 *one of the world's leaders in swimming pools per capita*   Dan Kois, "Iceland's Water Cure," *New York Times Magazine*, April 19, 2016; Egill Bjarnason, "Swimming with the Locals: 10 of Iceland's Best Pools," *Lonely Planet*, August 2017.

44 *a group of thirty ocean swimmers preparing for a swim*
"President of Iceland Takes Ocean Swim," *Iceland Review*,
October 2, 2017.

48 *one-fifth of the world's puffins come back*   Hálfdán
Helgason, "Survival of Atlantic Puffins (*Fratercula arctica*) in
Vestmannaeyjar, Iceland during Different Life Stages," paper
published for the Faculty of Life and Environmental Sciences at
the University of Iceland, 2011, pdfs.semanticscholar.org/50b8/
861d211d54daf9245a1ecod36d2167e828fb.pdf.

This paper references numerous other scientific sources for further
reading.

57 *Reading the Australian philosopher Damon Young*   Damon
Young, "Why Swimming Is Sublime," *Guardian*, February 7,
2014.

WELL-BEING

5. The Water Cure

67 *Benjamin Franklin swam daily in the Thames*   Kate Stanton,
"American Politicians Who Loved Skinnydipping," United
Press International, August 20, 2012; Philip Hoare, review of
*Downstream: A History and Celebration of Swimming the River
Thames* by Caitlin Davies, *Guardian*, April 24, 2015.

67 *one writer has called "a mess of maladies"*   Adee Braun, "The
Historic Healing Power of the Beach," *Atlantic*, August 29, 2013.

67 *water therapy became big business*   W. Caleb McDaniel,
"Spreading the News about Hydropathy: How Did Americans
Learn to Stop Worrying and Trust the Water Cure?," paper
presented at the annual meeting of the Society for Historians of
the Early American Republic, Baltimore, MD, 2012, available in
Rice University's Digital Scholarship archive.

68 *a journal dedicated to the subject*   The motto of *The Water-Cure
Journal: Devoted to Physiology, Hydropathy, and the Laws of
Life* was "Wash and Be Healed." It was published between 1845
and 1862 and is available through an online database managed by
the International Association for the Preservation of Spiritualist

and Occult Periodicals, http://www.iapsop.com/archive/materials/water-cure_journal/.

68 *Cold water was proclaimed the sovereign remedy* "The Water Cure," *Boston Medical and Surgical Journal* (published by *New England Journal of Medicine*) 35, no. 18 (December 2, 1846).

68 *eight-volume* Hydropathic Encyclopedia, *published circa 1851* Russell Thacher Trall, *The Hydropathic Encyclopedia: A System of Hydropathy and Hygiene, in Eight Parts* (New York: Fowler and Wells, ca. 1851), available at the Schlesinger Library, Radcliffe Institute.

69 *Our trust in water as a cure-all goes back to the ancients* Roger Charlier et al. "The Healing Sea: A Sustainable Coastal Ocean Resource: Thalassotherapy," *Journal of Coastal Health* 25, no. 4 (July 2009).

69 *Called the "sailors' method"* A. Trousseau, *Lectures on Clinical Medicine, Delivered at the Hotel-Dieu, Paris*, vol. 35 (London: New Sydenham Society, 1868).

71 *Tanaka's lab has pioneered new research* Jason Gelt, "Making Waves: The Benefits of Swimming on Aging Populations," *University of Texas Education Magazine*, June 2014; Markham Heid, "Why Swimming Is So Good For You," *Time*, March 2, 2017.

72 *Tanaka and his co-researchers published a paper* Mohammad Alkatan et al., "Improved Function and Reduced Pain after Swimming and Cycling Training in Patients with Osteoarthritis," *Journal of Rheumatology* 43, no. 3 (March 2016).

73 *"If I don't swim, the pain grows"* Melissa Hung, "To Swim Is to Endure: On Living with Chronic Pain," *Catapult Magazine*, April 17, 2017.

73 *a swimming pool installed in the White House* "Brady Press Briefing Room," The White House Museum, http://www.whitehousemuseum.org/west-wing/press-briefing-room.htm (accessed April 13, 2019).

77 *Ohlone oral history tells us that Alcatraz* Troy Johnson, "We Hold the Rock: The Alcatraz Indian Occupation," National Park Service, www.nps.gov/alca/learn/historyculture/we-hold-the-rock.htm (last updated February 27, 2015); the NPS's extensive readings on

the island's history and culture also provided larger background
for this chapter, as did Jerry Lewis Champion Jr.'s *The Fading
Voices of Alcatraz* (Bloomington, IN: AuthorHouse, 2011).

77 *he published a sensational autobiography*   Roy Gardner's
Hellcatraz: The Rock of Despair; The Tomb of the Living Dead
was self-published in 1939.

78 *a recent study using computer modeling*   "Dummy Heads
Used to Fool Guards During the 1962 Alcatraz Breakout to Be
3D Scanned by the FBI Amid Fears the Originals Are Decaying
Quickly," *Daily Mail*, August 7, 2017.

79 *Anastasia Scott (no relation to the prisoner John Paul)*   "Girl,
17, Swims from Alcatraz: Crossing Easily Made by Soldier's
Daughter," *San Francisco Bay Chronicle*, October 18, 1933.

6. Seawater in Our Veins

82 *we have so-called gill slits*   "Acorn Worm Genome Reveals Gill
Origins of Human Pharynx," *Science Daily*, November 19, 2015.

82 *Seawater is so similar in mineral content to human blood
plasma*   Natalie Angier, "The Wonders of Blood," *New York
Times*, October 20, 2008; Burnside Foster, ed., *The St. Paul
Medical Journal*, vol. 7 (Saint Paul, MN: Ramsey County Medical
Society, 1905).

83 *Lynne Cox, the legendary open-water swimmer*   "Long, Cold
Swim," *New York Times*, August 9, 1987.

83 *Cox has participated in medical studies*   I spoke with Lynne Cox;
she also chronicles her experiences as a research subject in her
2016 book, *Swimming in the Sink*.

83 *Guðlaugur and Cox appeared in the same academic
journal*   Keating, William, "Arctic Swims." *Polar Record* 24,
no. 148 (1988).

83 *Cox's body fat has been estimated at 35 percent*   Rich Roberts,
"Orange County Woman Swims Bering Strait," *Los Angeles
Times*, August 8, 1987.

84 *"anticipatory thermogenesis": the creation of heat*   James
Butcher, "Lewis Gordon Pugh—Polar Swimmer," *Lancet*,
Medicine and Sport special issue, 366 (December 2005).

85 *Tanaka went back to Japan to study the* ama   Hirofumi Tanaka et al., "Arterial Stiffness of Lifelong Japanese Female Pearl Divers," *American Journal of Physiology Regulatory, Integrative and Comparative Physiology* 310 (March 2016), https://www .physiology.org/doi/pdf/10.1152/ajpregu.00048.2016; Laura Kiniry, "On the Job with Japan's Legendary Female Ama Divers," CNN, February 22, 2017.

85 *growing body of research on the therapeutic benefits*   Takeshi Matsui and Sho Onodera, "Cardiovascular Responses in Rest, Exercise, and Recovery Phases in Water Immersion," *Journal of Sports Medicine and Physical Fitness* 2, no. 4 (2013).

86 *one-hour head-out immersion in ninety-degree water* A. Mooventhan and L. Nivethitha, "Scientific Evidence-Based Effects of Hydropathy on Various Systems of the Body," *North American Journal of Medical Sciences* 6, no. 5 (May 2014).

86 *regular cold-water winter swimming significantly reduces tension*   P. Huttunen, L. Kokko, and V. Ylijukuri, "Winter Swimming Improves General Well-Being," *International Journal of Circumpolar Health* 63, no. 2 (2004).

87 *elite swimmers, unlike elite runners, can excel*   Gretchen Reynolds, "How Body Type May Determine Runners' and Swimmers' Destinies," *New York Times*, August 14, 2018.

87 *duck into the office of Dr. Shingo Kajimura*   I spoke with Kajimura at length about his work; additional information about his research publications are available from the University of California, San Francisco, https://profiles.ucsf.edu/shingo .kajimura#toc-id5.

91 *"Her eyelashes froze solid and she couldn't open them"*   Ram Barkai wrote about his experiences in Tyumen in "Done! Nothing Can Explain the Sense of Euphoria after Completing Such an Intimidating Challenge." *Siberian Times*, December 23, 2012, https://siberiantimes.com/sport/others/features/done-nothing-can-explain-the-sense-of-pride-and-euphoria-after-completing-such-an-intimidating-challenge/; I also spoke to Barkai by phone about his follow-up swims and the founding of the International Ice Swimming Association.

97 *John Aldridge, the lobsterman from Long Island*   Paul Tough, "A Speck in the Sea," *New York Times Magazine*, January 2, 2014.

98 *Thomas Nuckton, an intensive care specialist*   Nuckton has published several papers on the effects of cold-water swimming; see https://www.researchgate.net/scientific-contributions/9800957_Thomas_J_Nuckton.

98 *In a 2015 study of experienced ice-mile swimmers*   Beat Knechtle et al., "Ice Swimming and Changes in Body Core Temperature: A Case Study," *SpringerPlus*, August 5, 2015, https://doi.org/10.1186/s40064-015-1197-y.

7. Open Water, Meet Awe

101 *hundreds of swimmers gather*   Julia Baird, "Forget Calories. Exercise for Awe," *New York Times*, May 6, 2017.

102 *after experiencing awe, we are more likely to help others*   Melanie Rudd et al., "Awe Expands People's Perception of Time, Alters Decision Making, and Enhances Well-Being," *Psychological Science*, August 10, 2012.

107 *Deep breathing research is in its infancy*   Gretchen Reynolds, "Why Deep Breathing May Keep Us Calm," *New York Times*, April 5, 2017; Katherine Ellen Foley, "Scientists Finally Understand Why Deep Breathing Physically Reduces Stress," *Quartz*, March 31, 2017.

108 *"Swimming in water is the only state of being I know where I feel free"*   Lidia Yuknavitch, "I Will Always Inhabit the Water," *Literary Hub*, April 12, 2017, https://lithub.com/lidia-yuknavitch-i-will-always-inhabit-the-water/.

109 *Swimming is the second most popular recreational activity*   "Americans' Participation in Outdoor Recreation," National Survey on Recreation and the Environment, USDA Forest Service, Recreation, Wilderness, and Demographics Trends Research Group, http://www.srs.fs.usda.gov/trends/Nsre/Rnd1t13weightrpt.pdf (accessed April 13, 2019).

111 *"The Women could swim off to the Ship, & continue half a day in the Water"*   The Journals of Captain James Cook on his Voyages of Discovery, Volume III, Part One, The Voyage of

the *Resolution and Discovery, 1776-1780* (London: Cambridge
University Press, 1967), available on Google Books, https://books
.google.com/books?id=Ty4rDwAAQBAJ.

COMMUNITY

119 *In Baghdad, which has been called*   Alexander Smith, "Baghdad,
Iraq, Is Hottest City in World with Temperatures at 120 Degrees,"
NBC News, July 31, 2015.

120 *Saddam Hussein's royal palace and its outdoor pool*   Descriptions
of the pool and of Baghdad during this period were drawn from
interviews conducted with members of the Baghdad Swim Team,
and in consultation with maps, photographs, and news stories;
William Langewiesche's "Welcome to the Green Zone" (*Atlantic*,
November 2004) and Yochi Dreazen's "In Baghdad's Green
Zone, Echoes of U.S. Occupation (*Atlantic*, September 14, 2011)
were particularly helpful. I also spoke with David Guttenfelder,
a photographer for *National Geographic* who photographed
extensively in Iraq, for background.

120 *(eighty-one, by one count)*   Geoff Manaugh, "Saddam's Palaces:
An Interview with Richard Mosse," *BLDGBLOG*, May 27, 2009,
http://www.bldgblog.com/.

122 *he received an award from then Secretary of State Hillary
Clinton*   Jay Taylor received the 2009 Secretary of State Award
for Outstanding Volunteerism Overseas; see https://www.aafsw
.org/services/sosa/2009-winners.

8. Who Gets to Swim?

123 *Public pools first proliferated in big cities*   Background for
this chapter was drawn from Jeff Wiltse's *Contested Waters*
(Chapel Hill: University of North Carolina Press, 2007) and
interviews with Jay Taylor. Other sources include Linda Poon's
"Remembering Beaches as Battlegrounds for Civil Rights,
CityLab, June 21, 2017, and the New York City Department of
Parks and Recreation (https://www.nycgovparks.org/).

126 *Black children drown at a rate five times that of white
children*   From a 2014 study by the Centers for Disease Control

and Prevention, and the USA Swimming Foundation, which commissioned a 2017 University of Memphis health study on factors impacting swimming participation and competence, Julie Gilchrist and Erin M. Parker, "Racial/Ethnic Disparities in Fatal Unintentional Drowning among Persons Aged ≤29 Years—United States, 1999-2010," *Morbidity and Mortality Weekly* 63, no. 19 (May 16, 2014), https://www.cdc.gov/mmwr/preview/mmwrhtml/mm6319a2.htm; and C. Irwin et al., "Factors Impacting Swimming Participation and Competence Quantitative Report," USA Swimming Foundation, May 31, 2017, www.usaswimmingfoundation.org/docs/librariesprovider1/mas/factors-impacting-swimming-participation-and-competence-final-quantitative-report-may-31-2017.pdf.

129 *In 2008, five years after the US-led invasion* Steven Simon, "The Price of the Surge," *Foreign Affairs*, May/June 2008.

135 *The first municipal pool in England, the St. George's Baths* "A Chronology of English Swimming, c. 1750-1918," *International Journal of the History of Sport* 24, no. 5 (2007). Other dates and details about the NSS, early swim clubs, and significant events in English swimming are also described in this issue.

136 *the influential writer and social essayist Harriet Martineau* Harriet Martineau, *Health, Husbandry, and Handicraft* (London: Bradbury and Evans, 1861).

136 *The girlhood struggle with physical modesty* "Swimming and Gender in the Victorian World," *International Journal of the History of Sport* 24, no. 5 (2007).

136 *the centuries-old practice of "swimming a witch"* "The Swimming of Witches: Indicium Aquae," The Foxearth and District Local History Society, http://www.foxearth.org.uk/SwimmingOfWitches.html (accessed April 13, 2019).

138 *black-and-white photo taken in September 1906* *Swimming Lesson* [photograph], 1906, Hulton Archive, Getty Images, https://www.gettyimages.fr/detail/photo/swimming-lesson-photo/HE3155-001.

138 *Every year, 372,000 people die* This and other statistics in this chapter are sourced from the World Health Organization,

Global Report on Drowning: Preventing a Leading Killer,
2014, https://www.who.int/violence_injury_prevention/
global_report_drowning/en/.

139 *some research that shows parents are less attentive* Perry Klass,
"Keeping Children Safe at the Beach or Pool," *New York Times,*
June 11, 2018.

10. Chaos and Order

147 *documentaries about transgender swimmers and autistic
swimmers* *The Swimming Club*, directed by Cecilia Golding
and Nick Finegan (London: British Film Institute in association
with Dazed Digital, 2016), is about the Trans and Gender Non-
Conforming Swimming Group in London, and *Swim Team*,
directed by Lara Stolman (Brooklyn: Argot Pictures, 2017), is
about a New Jersey team of swimmers on the autism spectrum.

COMPETITION

153 *"Salmon fry: five to ten weeks old and swimming"* The Nature
Conservancy, *A Landscape Risk Assessment Framework for
Salmon,* July 30, 2015, https://www.conservationgateway.org/
ConservationByGeography/NorthAmerica/UnitedStates/alaska/
scak/Documents/Landscape_Risk_Framework_July_2015.pdf.

154 *aboriginal peoples along the northwest coast of North
America* Kira Gerwing and Timothy McDaniels, "Listening to
the Salmon People: Coastal First Nations' Objectives Regarding
Salmon Aquaculture in British Columbia," *Society and Natural
Resources* 19, no. 3 (2006).

155 *to be ignorant of "either letters or swimming"* H. N. Couch,
"Swimming among the Greeks and Barbarians," *Classical Journal*
29, no. 8 (May 1934).

155 *"great numbers of the barbarians"* Herodotus, *Herodotus,*
translated from the Greek by William Beloe (Philadelphia: Thomas
Wardle, 1839).

155 *swimming's great value as a martial art* Historical references to
ancient art, the Greeks and Romans, and the shift from military
to athletic focus can be found in Anonymous's *The Science of*

Swimming (New York, 1849) and Stathis Avramidis's "World Art on Swimming," *International Journal of Aquatic Research and Education* 5 (2011).

156 *Pugh stood on the edge of an Arctic iceberg* I spoke with Lewis Pugh and consulted written accounts of his polar swims.

11. The Splash and Dash

159 *At forty-one, she was the oldest Olympic swimmer in history* I interviewed Dara Torres at length about her long career and about this swim in particular. Footage of her Beijing 50-meter final can be found at http://www.youtube.com/watch?v=IJxFvVUonso.

160 *Fast-twitch muscle fibers, which supply* T. R. Henwood, S. Riek, and D. R. Taaffe, "Strength Versus Muscle Power-Specific Resistance Training in Community-Dwelling Older Adults," *Journals of Gerontology: Biological Sciences and Medical Sciences* 63 (2008).

160 *current male and female world record holders* For FINA 50-meter-pool world records as of November 23, 2018, see http://www.fina.org/sites/default/files/wr_50m_nov_23_2018.pdf.

162 *In the first modern Olympic Games* Sources for this chapter include Bill Mallon and Ture Widlund, *The 1896 Olympic Games: Results for All Competitors in All Events, with Commentary* (Jefferson, NC: McFarland, 1998); and Olympic Studies Centre, *Aquatics: History of Swimming at the Olympic Games*, reference document prepared for the International Olympic Committee, March 2015, https://stillmed.olympic.org/AssetsDocs/OSC%20Section/pdf/QR_sports_summer/Sports_Olympiques_natation_eng.pdf.

163 *Charlotte "Eppie" Epstein founded the Women's Swimming Association* Linda Borish, "Charlotte Epstein: 1884-1938," *Jewish Women's Archive Encyclopedia*, https://jwa.org/encyclopedia/article/Epstein-Charlotte (accessed April 13, 2019). See also the International Swimming Hall of Fame, ishof.org/charlotte-epstein-(usa).html.

164 *American Association of Park Superintendents published bathing suit regulations* Benjamin Marcus describes the evolution of

men's swimwear in *Surfing: An Illustrated History of the Coolest Sport of All Time* (Minneapolis, MN: MVP Books, 2013).

165 *Ederle was Epstein's ultimate success story* For more about Ederle, read Glenn Stout's *Young Woman and the Sea* (New York: Houghton Mifflin Harcourt, 2009).

166 *Lloyd's of London took bets on Ederle* George Witte, "Freak Insurance Issued by Lloyd's," *Springfield News-Leader*, July 25, 1926.

166 *Women's Swimming Association's "girl swim stars"* "Local Mermaids Favored for Titles," *New York Times*, January 30, 1927; "Miss Epstein to Head Women's Swim Club," *New York Times*, November 14, 1928; "Intensive Preparations for Olympic Games Planned by Women's Swimming Association," *New York Times*, November 28, 1931; "Back-Stroke Record Broken by Kompa Sisters in 'Gertrude Ederle Day' Meet," *New York Times*, August 9, 1936; "Three Titles Won by Women's Swimming Association Stars in A. A .U. Meet," *New York Times*, July 10, 1938.

169 *The international space station can travel* The ISS needs to travel at least 17,500 miles per hour, or about 5 miles a second, to remain in orbit; see "Space Shuttle and International Space Station," Kennedy Space Center, http://www.nasa.gov/centers/kennedy/about/information/shuttle_faq.html#14 (accessed April 13, 2019).

169 *It's less than a flap of a hummingbird's wing* A hummingbird's wings average sixty to eighty beats per second (though it can beat much faster in bursts while diving; "Photo Ark," *National Geographic*, https://www.nationalgeographic.org/projects/photo-ark/ [accessed April 13, 2019]); a blink of an eye lasts about a tenth of a second (Ben Mauk, "Why Do We Blink?," *Live Science*, October 24, 2012).

12. How to Swim Like an Assassin

173 *She never visualized winning anything but gold* I spoke with Ledecky's coach, Bruce Gemmell, and consulted numerous print and television interviews Ledecky gave to the *Washington Post* and others. (Despite repeated requests for interviews through

Stanford University and eventual professional representatives, Ledecky declined to be interviewed for this book, citing time constraints.)

176   *"so I could broaden my mind and believe"*   Tim Layden, "After Rehabilitation, the Best of Michael Phelps May Lie Ahead," *Sports Illustrated*, November 5, 2015; and Jon Fortt, "The 'Craziest' Thing Michael Phelps Did to Be the Greatest Swimmer of All Time," CNBC, March 5, 2017. (Despite requests for interviews to Phelps's professional representatives, I was never able to speak with him directly.)

13. Sharks and Minnows

180   *home video evidence of Ledecky*   Dave Sheinin, "How Katie Ledecky Became Better at Swimming Than Anyone Is at Anything," *Washington Post*, June 24, 2016, including interactive graphics and video.

184   *Established in 1970, US Masters now has*   US Masters Swimming, https://www.usms.org (accessed April 13, 2019).

14. Ways of the Samurai

192   *writings dating back hundreds of years describe samurai swimming*   Background information for this chapter was drawn from interviews with numerous members of the Japan Swimming Federation and the national committee on *Nihon eiho*, and with practitioners of the art. I also consulted several invaluable texts, in particular *Swimming in Japan* (Tokyo: International Young Women and Children's Society, 1935); Matthew De George's *Pooling Talent: Swimming's Greatest Teams* (Lanham, MD: Rowman & Littlefield, 2014); and Antony Cummins's *Samurai and Ninja: The Real Story Behind the Japanese Warrior Myth that Shatters the Bushido Mystique* (North Clarendon, VT: Tuttle Publishing, 2015). Scholarly articles include Andreas Niehaus's "Swimming into Memory: The Los Angeles Olympics (1932) as Japanese *lieu de mémoire*," *Sport in Society* 14, no. 4 (2011); Atsunori Matsui, Toshiaki Goya, and Hiroyasu Satake, "The History and Problem of Swimming Education in Japan," paper presented at the International Aquatic History Symposium and

Film Festival, Fort Lauderdale, FL, May 2012. Midori Ishibiki shared a personally translated copy of Setsuzo Mikami's century-old history of *Nihon eiho, Stories at Random about Japanese Swimming.*

193   *a combined team that included England, Australia, and the United States*   Per interviews with Midori Ishibiki and Masaaki Imamura.

195   *a "speeded-up form" of* hira-oyogi   From *Swimming in Japan* (Tokyo: International Young Women and Children's Society, 1935): Tsuruta writes on Japanese tradition and the breaststroke.

196   *Butterfly, strangely enough, evolved from breaststroke*   Marie Doezema, "The Murky History of the Butterfly Stroke," *New Yorker*, August 11, 2016.

198   *In a Japanese television report, a samurai lowers*   This *Sports Japan* segment, shared with me by Midori Ishibiki, is also available at http://www.youtube.com/watch?v=WwDvJeP4WOg.

200   *comes directly from the Nojima ryu*   Per interviews with Midori Ishibiki.

207   *Cundy is the only non-Japanese person*   I was introduced to Tony Cundy by Midori Ishibiki, who confirmed his status.

209   *"The fuller sense of self we have"*   Brandon Ambrosino interviews Damon Young in "Exercise Can Make You More Thoughtful, Creative, and Ethical," *Vox*, February 12, 2015.

210   *"Real swimming is using the whole body"*   Sawai Atsuhiro describes the ideals of samurai swimming in "My Introduction to Bujutsu," which appeared in the Summer 2005 issue of the Shudokan Martial Arts Association newsletter, https://www.smaa-hq.com/articles.php?articleid=16.

FLOW

216   *"the state in which people are so involved"*   Mihaly Csikszentmihalyi describes this theory in his book *Flow: The Psychology of Optimal Experience* (New York: Harper & Row, 1990).

217 *Byron was obsessed with swimming* Merrell Noden, "Lord of the Waterways," *Sports Illustrated*, May 25, 1987.

217 *"I delight in the sea"* Thomas Medwin, *Conversations of Lord Byron* (Princeton, NC: Princeton Legacy Library, 2015).

218 *what the cultural historian Jacques Barzun once described* Jacques Barzun, "Byron and the Byronic," *Atlantic*, August 1953.

15. A Religious Exercise

220 *has defined zone and flow* Robert Nideffer, "Getting into the Optimal Performance State," https://www.epstais.com/articles/optimal.pdf (accessed April 13, 2019).

220 *The neuropsychologist David Eagleman has determined* Eagleman has written extensively on this subject, including the paper "Does Time Really Slow Down during a Frightening Event?," with Chess Stetson and Matthew P Fiesta, *PLoS ONE* 2, no. 12 (2007).

222 *"Being around water provides"* Wallace Nichols, *Blue Mind* (New York: Little, Brown, 2014).

222 *with his "great whalelike bulk"* Oliver Sacks writes about his lifelong love affair with swimming in "Water Babies," *New Yorker,* May 26, 1997.

223 *Cognitive scientists have shown that water sounds* "It's True: The Sound of Nature Helps Us Relax," *Science Daily*, March 30, 2017, describes a new University of Sussex study led by Cassandra Gould; Laura Schiff and Hollis Kline, "Water's Wonders," *Psychology Today*, September 2001.

224 *Though Einstein could not swim* Albert Einstein, *The Travel Diaries of Albert Einstein* (Princeton, NJ: Princeton University Press, 2018).

227 *A rural New Hampshire farm was home* See Maxine Kumin's website, https://maxinekumin.com, and the Poetry Foundation, https://www.poetryfoundation.org (accessed April 13, 2019).

16. The Liquid State

232 *Phelps was diagnosed with ADHD*   See Phelps's book, *No Limits: The Will to Succeed* (New York: Free Press, 2008), written with Alan Abrahamson.

233 *Bill Clinton once told PBS*   Bill Clinton, interviewed by Judy Woodruff, "Bill Clinton's Advice for His Wife on Running for President: 'Get Healthy,'" PBS *NewsHour*, September 23, 2013, https://www.pbs.org/newshour/nation/bill-clintons-advice-for-his-wife-on-running-for-president-get-healthy.

17. From One Swimmer to Another

248 "the color of there seen from here"   Rebecca Solnit, *A Field Guide to Getting Lost* (New York: Viking Penguin, 2005).